Molecular Basis of Human Nutrition

LIFELINES

MOLECULAR BASIS OF HUMAN NUTRITION

■ Tom Sanders and Peter Emery
Department of Nutrition and Dietetics,
King's College London, UK

Taylor & Francis
Taylor & Francis Group
LONDON AND NEW YORK

First published 2003 by Taylor & Francis
11 New Fetter Lane, London EC4P 4EE

Simultaneously published in the USA and Canada
by Taylor & Francis Inc,
29 West 35th Street, New York, NY 10001

Taylor & Francis is an imprint of the Taylor & Francis Group

© 2003 Taylor & Francis

Typeset in 11/13pt Perpetua by Graphicraft Limited, Hong Kong
Printed and bound in Great Britain by TJ International Ltd, Padstow, Cornwall

Every effort has been made to ensure that the advice and information in this book is true
and accurate at the time of going to press. However, neither the publisher nor the authors
can accept any legal responsibility or liability for any errors or omissions that may be
made. In the case of drug administration, any medical procedure or the use of technical
equipment mentioned within this book, you are strongly advised to consult the
manufacturer's guidelines.

British Library Cataloguing in Publication Data
A catalogue record for this book is available from the British Library

Library of Congress Cataloging in Publication Data
A catalog entry has been requested

ISBN 0-415-29917-9 (hbk)
ISBN 0-748-40753-7 (pbk)

CONTENTS

SERIES EDITOR'S PREFACE

Teaching programmes in universities now are generally arranged in collections of discrete units. These go under various names such as units, modules, or courses. They usually stand alone as regards teaching and assessment but, as a set, comprise a programme of study. Usually around half of the units taken by undergraduates are compulsory and effectively define a 'core' curriculum for the final degree. The arrangement of teaching in this way has the advantage of flexibility. The range of options over and above the core curriculum allows the student to choose the best programme for her or his future.

The Lifeline series provides a selection of texts that can be used at the undergraduate level for subjects optional to the main programme of study. Each volume aims to cover the material at a depth suitable to a particular level or year of study, with an amount of material appropriate to around one-quarter of the undergraduate year. The concentration of life science subjects in the Lifeline series reflects the fact that it is here that individual topics proliferate.

Suggestions for new subjects and comments on the present volumes in the series are always welcomed and should be addressed to the series editor.

John Wrigglesworth
King's College London

PREFACE

This book is aimed at first or second year undergraduates, or taught master's students, who are studying nutrition as part of a degree in molecular life sciences, health sciences or medicine, including single honours nutrition students. It is intended to supplement the larger nutrition textbooks with greater emphasis on the molecular and metabolic basis of nutrition. It focuses on the biochemical functions of the essential nutrients and the physiological consequences of deficient and excessive intakes. These are described within the context of normal human diets and the requirements for health. Consideration is also given to the other biologically active materials within foods, and to the role of diet in multifactorial diseases. The book focuses on human nutrition, although there are instances where comparisons with, or examples from, the nutrition of other mammalian species will be mentioned to help in the understanding of basic nutritional principles.

It is assumed that readers will have studied, or will be studying concurrently, first year undergraduate modules in general biochemistry and mammalian physiology. The book is based on our experience of many years of research and teaching in nutrition.

Tom Sanders and Peter Emery
King's College London

ACKNOWLEDGEMENTS

The authors are grateful to Dr John Wrigglesworth for his comments on the manuscript and to Mila Sanders for help with the illustrations and for checking the manuscript.

INTRODUCTION

What we eat has an enormous impact on our health. Nutritional deficiencies in developing countries are responsible for the major causes of blindness and brain damage worldwide, contribute to high rates of childhood mortality and affect the capacity of adults to work. On the other hand, in the economically developed areas of the world, obesity is an increasing threat to health and the composition of food eaten has a strong influence on the risk of many chronic diseases such as stroke, coronary heart disease, cancer and dental caries. Recent mass outbreaks of food poisoning and the apparent transmission of bovine spongiform encephalopathy (BSE) to humans have highlighted how important a role food plays in the spread of new diseases. In this book, we attempt to explain the molecular basis of human nutrition by outlining the role of nutrients in the body, the consequences of deficient and excessive intakes, the mechanisms involved in diet-related disease and other hazards associated with food intake.

■ 1.1 WHAT IS NUTRITION?

Nutrition can be defined as the process by which living matter acquires substances called nutrients for growth, repair and energy. However, this narrow definition does not adequately describe the effects of food intake on metabolic processes, as food also contains non-nutritive material. Non-nutritive material is more prevalent in food of plant origin. Some of these compounds exert pharmacological effects (e.g. caffeine in coffee). Indeed, many drugs are derived from plants. However, the body has the capacity to adapt to metabolize a wide variety of chemicals and generally converts them into forms which can be excreted. The science of human nutrition is better defined as being concerned with understanding the effects of food on the human body in both health and disease.

Nutrients and non-nutritive materials consist of chemical entities. The contribution a food makes to intake is a function of (i) the concentration of the chemical entity in the food; (ii) the amount consumed; and (iii) the frequency of consumption. For example, parsley contains a high concentration of vitamin C (approximately 1mg/g) but is only consumed in small amounts (no more than 5 g/serving) occasionally (perhaps once a week), and therefore only contributes small amounts to the total weekly intake ($1 \times 5 \times 1 = 5$ mg/week). On the other hand, potatoes contain moderate amounts of vitamin C (0.15 mg/g) but are consumed frequently (say 4 occasions/week) in substantial amounts (typically 150 g/portion) so contribute substantially to total intake (90 mg/week). In order that comparisons can be made between individuals of different size, an adjustment can be made by dividing the intake by body weight. The term dietary exposure is used to express the intakes and this is normally expressed in relation to body weight:

Nutritional value = quantity × quality

$$\text{Dietary exposure} = \frac{(\text{food chemical}) \times \text{daily food consumption}}{\text{body weight}}$$

Some compounds have the capacity to accumulate in the body. In the case of nutrients that can be stored, such as vitamin A, this means that a regular intake is not necessary. For example, 100 g of lamb's liver contains about 30,000 retinol equivalents (r.e.) which are sufficient to meet the requirements of an individual for about a month. On the other hand, a regular, low intake of a non-nutritive compound that accumulates in the body could be cumulatively toxic. For example, some fat-soluble pesticides such as DDT can accumulate in body fat. Furthermore, some compounds can accumulate up the food chain (Figure 1.1) with the highest levels being found in carnivorous animals at the top of the food chain. For example, the liver of the polar bear contains very high concentrations of vitamin A and whale meat can contain very high levels of toxic heavy metals.

Fat-soluble nutrients and contaminants which are not readily excreted accumulate up the food chain

Nutrients can be subdivided into macronutrients (protein, fat, carbohydrates and the major minerals Na, K, Ca, Mg, Cl, P) and micronutrients (vitamins and trace minerals) which are needed in smaller amounts (mg or µg/d). The main role of macronutrients is to supply energy and structural material (proteins, membranes, teeth and bones) and to make compounds needed for normal metabolism (hormones, enzymes etc), whereas the main role of micronutrients is to act as cofactors required for normal metabolism. The specific roles of each nutrient and the consequences of deficiencies are discussed in the ensuing chapters.

• **Figure 1.1** Chemicals and fat-soluble nutrients can accumulate up the food chain

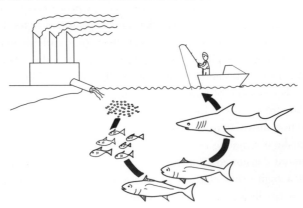

• **Figure 1.2** Relationship between decreasing intakes of vitamin A and indices of deficiency

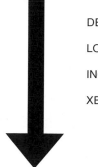

INCREASING DEFICIENCY

DEPLETED LIVER STORES

LOW BLOOD LEVELS

INCREASED RISK OF INFECTION

XEROPHTHALMIA
— NON BLINDING
— BLINDING

■ 1.2 ESTIMATION OF NUTRIENT REQUIREMENTS

The aim of the process of estimating nutrient requirements is to prevent harm arising from a lack of the nutrient, but at the same time to safeguard against adverse effects arising from excessive intakes. The assessment of nutrient requirements depends heavily upon the criteria used. This is well illustrated by an experiment conducted in rats fed varying intakes of vitamin A. It was possible to prevent the major signs of vitamin deficiency (blindness, sterility, altered cell division) with 5 µg/d of vitamin A, but greater amounts were required for a normal visual threshold (8 µg/d), while for normal liver storage of the vitamin an intake of 24 µg/d was required. Even higher intakes are required for optimum growth and reproduction. The same pattern can be seen in humans by observing the stages of vitamin A deficiency (Figure 1.2). Tissue stores become depleted and an increased risk of infection occurs before clinical signs and symptoms of deficiency are observed.

> Clinical signs are what can be observed whereas symptoms are what the patient reports

The three main methods used to estimate human nutrient requirements are: 1) determination of the amount required to prevent or cure a deficiency disease, 2) determination of the amount required to maintain a nutrient balance, and 3) determination of the amount needed to optimize biochemical processes that are dependent on the nutrient. Each of these methods can give different results. Clinical deficiencies are usually only apparent when deficiency is severe, and so estimates of requirements using this method tend to be lower than for the other methods.

The amount that is sufficient to cure or prevent a deficiency disease is sometimes referred to as the **minimal requirement**; however, an intake that is adequate to prevent or cure the classical deficiency disease but still results in functional impairments is regarded as suboptimal. This is well illustrated by reference to vitamin C. Experiments carried out on a small number of conscientious objectors to military service in the Second World War in Sheffield showed that a daily intake of 10 mg of vitamin C was sufficient to prevent and cure the deficiency disease scurvy. However, an intake of 20 mg/d was required to support normal wound healing. Moreover, later studies conducted on a large number of subjects showed that an intake of 30 mg/d decreased the risk of gingivitis (inflammation of the gums). It should be noted that one of the

> The amount of a nutrient required to prevent/cure a deficiency disease is regarded as the minimal requirement

features of scurvy is inflammation of the gums, which become purplish and spongy and bleed. Consequently an intake of 10 mg/d of vitamin C is regarded as suboptimal and higher intakes are needed to maintain optimal wound healing and protection against gingivitis.

The second method is to determine the intake that will allow the body to maintain a balance between intake and utilization. However, this approach has some limitations because the body can adapt to low intakes of some nutrients, and thus maintain a balance over quite a wide range of intakes. This is well illustrated by a study of experimental scurvy conducted on prisoners in the Iowa State Penitentiary, USA. The subjects were put on a vitamin C-deficient diet and injected with a radioactively labelled form of the vitamin so that the rate of utilization of vitamin C and the size of the body pool could be estimated. It was observed that as the body pool of vitamin C became depleted, so the rate of its utilization decreased such that the turnover of vitamin C was 3 per cent of the body pool size: when the pool size was 1,500 mg the rate of turnover was about 30 mg/d, whereas when the pool size was 300 mg the turnover was only 9 mg/d. Similar adaptations occur on low intakes of protein, where the catabolism of amino acids to urea is suppressed, and on low energy intakes, where energy expenditure decreases. Thus for vitamin C the Reference Nutrient Intake (RNI–see p.5) is based on the amount needed to maintain an adequate pool size, as indicated by the circulating concentration. However, it can be argued that intake is adequate only when it saturates the body pool (in the case of a nutrient where excess intakes are excreted) or when it enables storage of the nutrient in the body. For example, estimates of the dietary requirement for vitamin A are based on the capacity of the liver to store more than 20 µg/g.

The third method uses functional indices that relate to the biochemical role of the nutrient. This approach can be applied to many vitamins which are coenzymes in metabolic reactions. For example, a deficiency of vitamin B_{12} results in elevations of plasma homocysteine and methyl malonic acid concentrations because the vitamin is a cofactor for methionine synthase and methyl malonyl mutase. Consequently, the amount of vitamin B_{12} required to normalize plasma concentrations of these metabolites can be used to assess requirements.

A major weakness of these three methods is that they do not take into account potential health benefits/risks that may result from intakes greater than those that fulfil the criteria for assessing requirements. For example, an increased intake of 400 µg/d folic acid on top of the normal dietary intake in the first trimester of pregnancy has been shown to decrease the risk of a woman giving birth to a child with a neural tube defect. On the other hand, high intakes of folic acid may increase the risk of spontaneous abortion in a pregnancy already affected by a neural tube defect. However, women who give birth to infants with neural tube defects do not show any of the classical signs of folate deficiency, and their dietary intake does not differ from women who give birth to healthy babies. One interpretation is that folic acid is exerting a pharmacological effect in those susceptible to having an affected pregnancy. It also raises the question as to whether folic acid really prevents neural tube defects or whether it makes the abortion of an affected foetus more likely. It therefore raises the issue of whether all women should be advised to take additional folic acid in early pregnancy. Questions such as these can only be resolved by large controlled trials where subjects are allocated either an active or placebo

• **Figure 1.3** Influence of folic acid supplementation on the outcome of pregnancy (*Source*: adapted from Berry *et al.*, 1999)

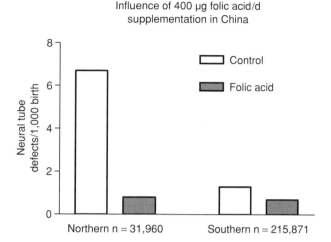

Influence of 400 µg folic acid/d
supplementation in China

treatment and the outcome observed. The results of such trials showed that folic acid supplementation improved the outcome of pregnancy (i.e. that there were fewer pregnancies affected by neural tube defects) but that the protective effect was greater where the habitual intake of folate was lowest.

■ 1.2.1 DIETARY REFERENCE VALUES

The generic term Dietary Reference Values (DRV) is used to describe a series of values which relate to estimates of the nutritional needs of groups of individuals and populations. They include the following: Estimated Average Requirement (EAR), Recommended Dietary Allowances (RDA), Reference Nutrient Intake (RNI), Lower Reference Nutrient Intake (LRNI), Safe Intake and Tolerable Upper Intake Level. DRVs are also used to describe the desirable proportions of food energy derived from fat, saturated fatty acids and carbohydrate, and the desirable intake of dietary fibre in order to prevent diet-related disease (the scientific basis for these recommendations is discussed in Chapter 9).

> Dietary Reference Values (DRV) is a generic term used to describe estimates of nutritional needs and dietary recommendations for groups of individuals and populations

The EAR is generally based on the amount that prevents deficiency and normalizes physiological and biochemical processes associated with a lack of the nutrient, as described above. However, for some nutrients deficiency disease is unknown among individuals following self-selected diets, so estimates of Safe Intake are made on the basis of the intakes in populations that are in good health (e.g. for vitamin E).

There is significant variation between individuals in nutrient requirements. Consequently, when setting the RNI or RDA, which are supposed to cover the nutrient requirements of almost all individuals, an allowance for individual variability is added on to EAR to ensure that the needs of individuals with above average requirements are met. The exception to this rule is for food energy where a positive energy balance would lead to weight gain. It should be noted that the available experimental data may not always give an accurate estimate of the true variability because it is often based on observations of a small number of healthy young subjects.

The assumption underlying the estimation of nutrient requirements is that the distribution of individual requirements within a population follows a normal distribution

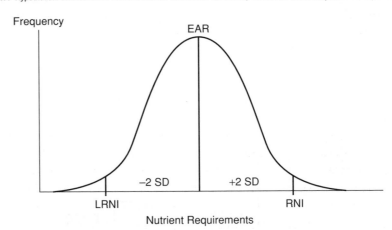

• **Figure 1.4** Hypothetical distribution of nutrient intakes taken from the Dietary Reference Values Report

(Figure 1.4). Thus there will be equal numbers of subjects with requirements below and above the EAR. In a normal distribution, adding 1.96 times the standard deviation to the mean value embraces all values except for the top 2.5 per cent of the population. The RNI is usually estimated by adding 2 standard deviations to the EAR (2 is an approximation of 1.96). This means that RNI is estimated to meet the requirements of 97.5 per cent of the population. There are, however, a few exceptions where this approach is not used, particularly where the nutrient is relatively toxic in excess (e.g. vitamin A). RNIs are often estimated in relation to body weight: the RNI for different age groups can be estimated by multiplying the RNI expressed in mg nutrient/kg body weight by the average body weight for each age group. For some nutrients, RNIs are expressed in relation to energy intake, for example in mg/kJ. This is because the requirement is linked to energy expenditure (for example, for thiamin, riboflavin and niacin). Additional allowances are also made for pregnancy and lactation.

Genetic and environmental factors cause variations in requirements. Gene polymorphisms are common variations in the gene encoding for a protein that result in altered but not entirely defective functioning of that protein. For example, about 10 per cent of the population carry the C677T polymorphism for the enzyme methyltetrahydrofolate reductase (MTHFR), which is a critical enzyme in folate metabolism, catalysing the conversion of 5, 10-methylene-tetrahydrofolate to 5-methyl-tetrahydrofolate. The MTHFR C677T polymorphism decreases MTHFR activity and thus increases the rate of utilization of plasma folate. There are also common polymorphisms of the 1, 25 $(OH)_2$ vitamin D receptor which influence sensitivity to vitamin D.

Environmental effects on nutrient requirements include factors such as stress, alcohol intake and cigarette smoking. For example, cigarette smoking increases the rate at which vitamin C is used by the body and consequently smokers have a higher requirement for the vitamin than non-smokers. Parasitic infestations (such as malaria, hookworm, giardiasis) which are common in many developing countries can also affect requirements because they either interfere with the absorption of nutrients or accelerate the rate at which the nutrients are used or lost from the body. Giardiasis is a common intestinal parasitic infection caused by the amoeba *Giardia lamblia*. It is prevalent in developing countries and results in decreased absorption of fat-soluble vitamins, particularly β-carotene (provitamin A). Infestation with hookworm, which is also prevalent in developing countries, results in an increased loss of iron due to bleeding into the gut. Malaria, which is a major public health problem in tropical countries, causes an increased turnover of red blood cells and, therefore, increases the requirement for nutrients associated with blood formation (iron, folate and vitamin B_{12}). Human immunodeficiency virus (HIV) infection can increase the risk of opportunistic infections of the gut that can result in the decreased absorption of several micronutrients.

For food labelling purposes, an average recommended daily allowance (RDA) figure is used. This is usually based on the RNI for an adult. However, there has been much confusion caused by the terms RDA and RNI. They were derived to be benchmarks by which to compare groups of individuals rather than to assess whether an individual has an adequate or inadequate intake of a nutrient. The terms are often misunderstood, for example, by journalists who suggest that the RNI is the minimum requirement. If an intake is above the RNI, then it is extremely unlikely that it will be inadequate. However, an individual may have an intake which is below the RNI but which is still perfectly adequate to meet their individual requirement. The Lower Reference Nutrient Intake (LRNI) is 2 standard deviations below the estimated average requirement. This can be used as a benchmark to assess whether an individual's habitual intake is likely to be in the range where their requirement may not be met.

Because the body requires a certain amount of a nutrient to function properly, it does not follow that greater amounts will necessarily improve health. Many nutrients can be purchased as supplements in health food shops and there have been cases of individuals consuming excessive amounts which have resulted in harm and even death, especially for vitamins A and D, and iron. Consequently, there has been a need to define safe upper limits for supplement use. The approach employed is to observe the lowest dose at which toxic effects occur and then allow a safety margin.

Small amounts of micronutrients are essential but excessive intakes can be toxic

■ 1.2.2 MEASUREMENTS OF TOXICITY

The Swiss sage Paracelsus recognized that plants could be foods, drugs or poisons, and that it was the dose that made the difference. Toxicity can be defined as the ability of a substance to cause harm when tested in isolation. All substances are toxic if sufficient amounts are consumed: whether a substance is a hazard (i.e. causes harm in practice) depends on the dose consumed, the timing and duration of exposure, the extent to which the compound can be metabolized and excreted and other factors that affect the sensitivity of the host such as age, gender and physiological state.

The nature of scientific investigation involves hypothesis testing, where a hypothesis is stated and an experiment designed to test the hypothesis. The statistical methods used in the testing of hypotheses are more robust at detecting significant differences than determining equivalence. Consequently, it is easier to demonstrate toxicity than to determine safety, which is the absence of potentially harmful effects. In order to assess toxicity, animals (usually mice and rats) are initially fed the test compound from high to low intakes in order to induce harmful effects. The lowest dose that induces adverse effects is then used to design long-term dietary exposure studies, often focusing on the organs where harm is observed in the acute test (this is called a target organ study). In these long-term studies, the aim is again to find the lowest intake of the compound that causes harm. This intake is termed the Lowest Adverse Effects Level (LOEL) and is expressed in mg/kg body weight. The intake below this is called the No Adverse Effects Level (NOEL). This figure is not likely to be precise but only an estimate depending on the number of dose levels used in the study.

In calculating a safe intake from the NOEL, several allowances are made to give a safety margin. An allowance is made for the variations in: 1) toxicokinetics, which are the properties which determine the delivery of the chemical to the target organ and the duration and extent of exposure, and 2) toxicodynamics, which are the properties which determine the response of the target organ to the chemical. In practice, the variability in toxicokinetics is usually taken as fourfold and that of toxicodynamics as two-and-a-half-fold. So if the NOEL value is divided by 10 (an approximation of the product of toxicokinetics and toxicodynamics) an estimated safe intake can be derived for the species in which the tests are conducted. However, if the results are to be extrapolated from animals to humans, a further safety factor is built in and this involves dividing the estimated safe intake by another factor of ten (again allowing for toxicokinetic and toxicodynamic variation) to yield an intake, usually expressed in mg/kg body weight. This is used as the basis for calculating the acceptable daily intake (ADI) (Figure 1.5).

• **Figure 1.5** Safety factors used in calculating acceptable daily intakes (ADI) from no observed effect level (NOEL) in animals

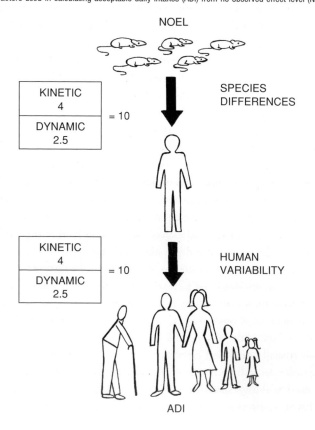

The ADI is defined as the amount of a chemical, expressed on a mg/kg body weight basis, that can be safely ingested each day over a lifetime. Daily intakes for men and women can then be calculated by multiplying by average body weight: the assumption generally used is that men weigh 60 kg and women weigh 50 kg (although this is considerably lower than actual average weights in the UK which are nearer 76 and 66 kg respectively). ADIs are set for food additives, which are intentionally added to food for a defined purpose during processing, and contaminants, which may be artificial or naturally occurring.

Variability in toxicokinetics and toxicodynamics is well illustrated by reference to the effects of alcohol. Anecdotal evidence suggests that women get drunk more easily than men and it has been proven that women are more likely to develop cirrhosis of the liver as a consequence of alcohol abuse. In men of all age groups and postmenopausal women, there is some oxidation of alcohol in the stomach prior to delivery to the liver (target organ) whereas this does not occur in women of reproductive age. Furthermore, because women contain more body fat than men, the distribution of alcohol in the body is different. This results in the same dose of alcohol/kg body weight, resulting in a higher blood alcohol concentration in women than men: these are all toxicokinetic effects. The effect blood alcohol has on the liver will depend on the size of the liver and its sensitivity to harmful effects: these are toxicodynamic effects. For example, the toxic effects of alcohol will be greater in an individual with an impaired capacity to metabolise alcohol or with some other pre-existing disorder such as chronic viral hepatitis. It is known that the livers of women are on average smaller than those of men and that they are more sensitive to the toxic effects of alcohol.

The risk of harm is regarded as neglible providing the ADI is not exceeded. If the ADI is occasionally exceeded, this is not of concern because of the large safety margin and because the ADI is set for long-term exposure. However, an ADI is not appropriate for compounds that can accumulate in the body. Several minerals such as arsenic, lead and mercury are cumulatively toxic, as are a large number of fat-soluble organochlorine compounds. Food of animal origin is generally not a source of toxic material unless the animal has accumulated a toxic substance from the food chain. As it is difficult to define safe intakes for such cumulatively toxic compounds, a Provisional Tolerable Weekly Intake (PTWI) expressed in mg/kg body weight is set. The PTWI is normally estimated by assessing how much of a given dose of the chemical is retained and estimating the rate of turnover of the compound. In some cases, the levels of compounds are irreducible (e.g. PCBs in oily fish) and so a more pragmatic view is taken which aims to set the PTWI as reasonably low as is achievable.

Non-nutritive material is more prevalent in foods of plant origin. Foods of plant origin are also the main source of potentially toxic material. For example, hydrogen cyanide is released by hydrolysis of cyanogenic glycosides, which are found in cassava, apricot kernels, linseed and butter beans. This is acutely toxic. Although there have been deaths resulting from individuals eating apricot kernels, acute cyanide toxicity is uncommon because cooking destroys most of the hydrogen cyanide and the small amounts present in apple pips are not sufficient to cause harm.

Plant foods contain a variety of potentially pharmacologically active substances, but food processing decreases dietary exposure and the effects are spread over a variety of receptors so that many of the pharmacological effects are balanced out. However, there can be synergistic interactions between pharmacologically active substances in food and drugs. For example, tyramine, which is a bacterial metabolite of the amino acid tryptophan, has a serious blood pressure raising effect in patients taking anti-depressant drugs that inhibit monoamine oxidase. Patients taking these drugs have to avoid sources of tyramine such as cheese, pickled fish and meat extracts. There are many such interactions with drugs and warnings are given on the data sheet for the drug. For example, terfenidine, a drug used to treat hay fever, was withdrawn from over-the-counter sales when it was discovered to interact with flavonoids in grapefruit juice and cause heart arrhythmias. On the other hand, some non-nutritive compounds may have beneficial effects on health by acting as antioxidants and cancer blocking agents (see Chapter 10).

■ 1.2.3 DIETARY GUIDELINES

Dietary guidelines have three primary aims: to provide a diet that meets the requirement for all nutrients; to avoid diet-related diseases such as obesity, cardiovascular disease, dental caries and cancer; and to prevent the transmission of foodborne diseases such as food poisoning and zoonoses including variant Creutzfeldt-Jakob disease. A detailed discussion of the risks and mechanisms relating to these conditions is given in Chapters 9 and 10. Dietary guidelines can be further divided into those which are aimed at the population, those that are given to caterers and the food industry, and those that are targeted at the individual. The latter are often known as food-based dietary guidelines. All dietary guidelines involve a risk/benefit analysis and to be successful they need to take into account normal human behaviour and recognize that the intake of food has an important social and cultural role.

The process by which dietary guidelines are derived is generally through consensus reports. These reports are written by committees of experts given specific terms of reference. Expert committees have been criticized because of the nature of the selection of their membership. Cronyism is the term used to describe the situation where committee members are selected from colleagues of one or two leading workers in the field. Stakeholders may also influence committee membership in order to ensure that their views are expressed. Experts who have links with industry, and lobby groups, are regarded as having a vested interest. This can lead to bias and the process has been criticized for lacking transparency and openness. An effort has been made to make the working of expert committees more open. However, this does tend to make the process more political and vulnerable to a different form of lobbying. More recently, the technique of systematic review has been applied to the development of dietary guidelines. In this process, strict rules are laid down concerning the admissibility of evidence. Systematic reviews were primarily developed for evaluating different treatment strategies and not for dealing with uncertainty. While this approach is an improvement, dietary guidelines should not be regarded as being written on tablets of stone.

The main focus of recent dietary guidelines has been to prevent obesity, cardiovascular disease, cancer and dental caries. All dietary guidelines advocate maintaining energy balance by matching energy intake with energy expenditure. Most dietary guidelines recommend that total fat intake should be decreased so that it provides between 25 and 35 per cent of energy, and that carbohydrate consumption should be increased to between 50 and 60 per cent of energy intake. These guidelines also recommend that intake of saturated fatty acids should not exceed 10 per cent of dietary energy, that intake of salt

Table 1.1 Dietary reference values from the UK Dietary Reference Values Report and the Eurodiet Consensus Conference

	UK DRV	EURODIET
Protein % energy	8–10	10–15
Fat % energy	35	<30
of which		
saturated fatty acids	10	<10
polyunsaturated fatty acids	6	4–8
trans fatty acids	<2	<2
Carbohydrates % energy	50	>55
of which non-milk extrinsic sugars	11	–
Dietary fibre g/d	18†	>25
Sodium chloride g/d	<6	<6

Note: †Expressed in terms on non-starch polysaccharide: approximately 20 g NSP is equivalent to 30 g dietary fibre.
Sources: Department of Health (1991; 1994); Proceedings of the European Conference (2000).

should be reduced to around 6 g/d and that intakes of dietary fibre (or non-starch polysaccharides) and potassium should be increased. Current UK DRVs and those proposed by the Eurodiet Consensus Conference are shown in Table 1.1. There is much dispute regarding the recommendations with regard to sugar. However, there is a consensus that the frequent consumption of sugar-containing snacks should be limited to no more than four eating occasions/day in order to help prevent dental caries. The scientific basis for these recommendations is given in Chapter 9.

Food-based dietary guidelines have been developed in order to translate the numerical DRVs into foods that make up the typical diet. These are often illustrated as a food pyramid or food on a plate showing the relative proportions of the major food groups that should make up a balanced diet. Replacing fatty meat and meat products, with lean meat and fish, is emphasized, as is using dairy products with a decreased fat content, and using vegetable oils sparingly in place of animal fats. In order to increase the intake of carbohydrate, an increased intake of starchy foods, preferably wholegrain cereals, is advocated rather than an increase in sugar consumption. One of the practical dietary guidelines has been to increase the recommended consumption of fruit and vegetables to five portions per day.

SUMMARY
- Nutrition is the effect of food intake on the human body in health and disease.
- Nutrient requirements vary according to age, gender, physiological state, genetic and environmental factors.
- Adaptation to low intakes of nutrients occurs.
- Excessive intakes of some vitamins and minerals can cause poisoning.
- Food contains both potentially toxic and beneficial non-nutritive material.
- Diet affects the risk of cardiovascular disease, cancer, diabetes and dental caries.
- Dietary Reference Value is the term used to describe estimates of the nutritional needs of groups of individuals and populations.

FURTHER READING

Department of Health (1991) *Dietary Reference Values for Food Energy and Nutrients for the United Kingdom. Report on Health and Social Subjects*, 41. London: HMSO.

'Nutrition and diet for healthy lifestyles in Europe: science and policy implications', Proceedings of the European Conference, Crete, Greece, May 18–20, 2000, *Public Health Nutr*, Apr 2001, 4(2A): 333–434.

Berry, R.J., Li Z., Erickson, J.D., Li, S., Moore, C.A., Wang, H., Mulinare, J., Zhao, P., Wong, L.Y., Gindler, J., Hong, S.Y., and Correa, A. (1999) 'Prevention of neural-tube defects with folic acid in China-China-US: Collaborative project for neural tube defect prevention IV.' *Eng. J. Med.* 341: 1485–90.

ENERGY

■ 2.1 ENERGY CONTENT OF FOODS

The human body obtains energy from four classes of nutrients: fats, carbohydrates, proteins and, for some people, alcohol. During digestion the macromolecules are hydrolysed to their monomers: fatty acids and glycerol from fats, monosaccharides from carbohydrates and amino acids from proteins. These monomers can then be taken up from the circulation by tissues and oxidised to generate ATP. Many tissues are able to utilize any or all of these molecules as fuel, although some show a marked preference or even an obligatory requirement for particular substrates (see Chapters 3, 4 and 5).

Energy can be obtained from fats, carbohydrates, proteins and alcohol

■ 2.1.1 GROSS ENERGY

Complete oxidation of these molecules yields carbon dioxide, water and oxides of nitrogen and sulphur, and liberates a certain amount of energy. The amount of energy generated by complete oxidation of a foodstuff is known as its gross energy content. This can be measured in a bomb calorimeter, in which the energy generated after igniting a known amount of the foodstuff in an atmosphere of pure oxygen is transferred to a known amount of water and the temperature rise in the water is measured. Precise determination of gross energy values in this way is relatively tedious, and most nutritional work nowadays utilizes a simpler instrument known as a ballistic bomb calorimeter. Here, the heat is transferred simply to the heavy metal casing of the combustion chamber, and the maximum temperature rise in the casing is measured. The instrument is calibrated by burning a similar amount of a standard substance, usually benzoic acid or sucrose, under the same conditions.

Gross energy is measured by bomb calorimetry

Representative values for the gross energy content of the major nutrients are shown in Table 2.1. If the nutrient composition of a foodstuff, or indeed a whole diet, is known then its gross energy content can be calculated as the algebraic sum of the gross energy contents of the individual nutrients.

Because the energy content of foods is measured by calorimetry, the results have generally been expressed in the traditional units of heat: calories. The word calorie has

Table 2.1 Gross energy content of major nutrients

	kJ/g	kcal/g
Carbohydrates		
Monosaccharides	15.7	3.75
Disaccharides	16.6	3.95
Polysaccharides	17.4	4.15
Polyols	8.3	2.00
Fats		
Average	39.1	9.3
Palmitic acid	27.5	6.1
Oleic acid	31.6	7.5
Linoleic acid	30.8	7.4
Proteins		
Average	22.9	5.4
Glycine	13.0	3.1
Phenylalanine	28.1	6.7
Ethanol	29.8	7.1

become so closely identified with this use in the public consciousness that it is now used colloquially as a synonym for the energy derived from food. However, from a scientific point of view it is important to recognise the equivalence of different forms of energy, and the accepted unit of energy is the joule. Thus, energy values are now always quoted in joules, although it is still useful in nutritional literature to quote equivalent values in calories as additional information; 1 calorie equals approximately 4.18 joules. Joules and calories are rather small units for measuring nutritionally significant amounts of food, so values are normally expressed in kilojoules (kJ) or kilocalories (kcal, sometimes abbreviated as Cal).

1 calorie = 4.18 joules

■ 2.1.2 DIGESTIBLE ENERGY

Digestible energy means the amount of energy from food actually absorbed by the body through the digestive tract. It is measured by subtracting the gross energy content of the faeces from the gross energy content of the food consumed.

Classic experiments by Atwater and others have measured the digestibility of pure nutrients. Alcohol is essentially 100 per cent absorbed. Glucose, sucrose and starch are at least 99 per cent digestible, which is why they are called available carbohydrates. Dietary fibre, or non-starch polysaccharide, is classically considered to have a digestibility of zero, although the fermentation of some non-starch polysaccharides in the large intestine means that a digestibility value of around 50 per cent may be more appropriate (see Chapter 4). The digestibility of fat is approximately 95 per cent, although there is some variation between different fats (see Chapter 5). The true digestibility of most animal proteins is also around 95 per cent, whereas the true digestibility of some plant proteins can be as low as 80 per cent. (See p. 39 in Chapter 3 on protein for a definition of true and apparent digestibility). Moreover, the addition of endogenous protein losses from the gut means that the apparent digestibility of mixed proteins in a typical Western diet is usually about 92 per cent, and it can be even lower in predominantly plant-based diets (see Chapter 3).

Digestible energy content can be predicted by applying these digestibility factors to the gross energy content of each component in a foodstuff or a diet. There is some evidence that large amounts of dietary fibre can inhibit the absorption of other components of a diet, but the effect appears to be very small.

■ 2.1.3 METABOLIZABLE ENERGY

Metabolizable energy is the amount of energy potentially available to the body to do work such as ATP synthesis. This is the conventional way of describing the energy content (or calorie content) of a diet or a foodstuff. It is measured by subtracting the gross energy content of the urine from the digestible energy intake. In humans, the difference between digestible and metabolizable energy values is due almost entirely to the energy content of the urinary urea. In other words, it arises because amino acids are not completely oxidized in the body to carbon dioxide, water and nitrogen oxides. Nitrogen is excreted in the form of urea, and this represents energy which is not available to the body. Hence although the gross energy value of most proteins is around 22.9 kJ/g (5.4 kcal/g), their metabolizable energy values are around 16.7 kJ/g (4.0 kcal/g).

For ruminant animals there is also a significant loss of energy in the breath in the form of methane which is produced during bacterial fermentation in the rumen, and this causes a somewhat greater difference between digestible energy and metabolizable energy values.

In practice, when constructing a table of food composition values or when analysing a diet, the metabolizable energy content is predicted from the amounts of protein, fat, alcohol and available carbohydrate present, multiplied by the average metabolizable energy value of each component. These average metabolizable energy values are often known as Atwater factors, and are shown in Table 2.2.

The energy values shown in tables of food composition are metabolizable energy values

■ 2.2 SOURCES OF ENERGY

Most foodstuffs contain a mixture of protein, fat and carbohydrate, as well as water. It is therefore somewhat misleading to refer to a particular foodstuff as a protein or a carbohydrate (except sugar), although it is appropriate in the case of oils and some fats. Since the Atwater factors for protein and carbohydrate are quite close to each other, the main determinant of the energy content per unit dry weight is the fat content. For pure fats this value will be 37 kJ/g (9 kcal/g), while for low fat foods it will be close to 17 kJ/g (4 kcal/g). In fact, even foods which are considered to have a high fat content, such as chocolate, peanuts and potato crisps, rarely exceed a value of 25 kJ/g (6 kcal/g).

The other major determinant of energy density (energy content per unit mass) is the water content. Foods with a high starch content often have a high water content as well.

Table 2.2 Average metabolizable energy values for macronutrients, or Atwater factors

	kJ/g	kcal/g
Available carbohydrate	16	3.75
Fat	37	9
Protein	17	4
Ethanol	29	7

Source: McCance and Widdowson's The Composition of Foods (2002).

Table 2.3 Contribution of macronutrients to food energy consumption in representative groups of countries

	% Energy from		
	Protein	*Carbohydrate*	*Fat*
Most affluent	11.5	53.0	35.7
Intermediate	10.4	67.5	22.1
Least affluent	10.1	74.7	15.2

Note: Data calculated from Food Balance Sheets (United Nations Food and Agriculture Organization).

The energy density of food is determined mainly by its fat and water contents

Thus bread is 40 per cent water and 50 per cent carbohydrate, giving an energy density of 9 kJ/g (2.2 kcal/g). Boiled rice is 70 per cent water and 6 kJ/g (1.4 kcal/g), potatoes are 80 per cent water and 3 kJ/g (0.7 kcal/g) and cabbage is 90 per cent water and 1 kJ/g (0.25 kcal/g).

The same analysis may be applied to the diet as a whole. Because of the dominant effect of water content, the most useful way of describing the proportions of the major nutrients in a diet is to refer to their contribution to the energy content of the diet. This also corrects for the effect of total energy intake, allowing qualitative comparisons between diets to be made. In particular, recommendations concerning the amount of fat in the diet are usually framed in terms of the proportion of energy coming from fat.

Table 2.3 shows the proportions of energy coming from the major nutrients in typical diets from different parts of the world, arranged in groups according to their affluence. The diets of people in the world's poorest countries tend to be dominated by carbohydrate, mainly from starchy staple foods. When economic constraints are removed, and people have access to a greater range of foods, they choose a much higher proportion of fat, while the amount of protein consumed varies over a much smaller range.

Clearly, energy requirements can be met by a wide range of diets. The specific requirement for protein appears to be met by most normal diets, with the possible exception of some diets of very low digestibility which may not meet the requirements of young infants in developing countries. Some tissues have an absolute requirement for glucose as a fuel (see Chapter 4), but the body can synthesize glucose from most amino acids or from glycerol. Since diets with a low carbohydrate content (such as the traditional Inuit diet) tend to be high in protein, dietary carbohydrate deficiency has never been observed. The minimum requirement for essential fatty acids is also small, amounting to around 1 per cent of dietary energy. In practical terms, however, very low fat diets are usually inadequate because of limited absorption of fat-soluble vitamins (see Chapter 5). Low fat, high carbohydrate diets also tend to be very bulky, particularly as they are likely to have a high water content. Cases have been reported where infants are unable to consume enough of such a bulky diet to meet their energy requirements, leading to protein–energy malnutrition.

■ 2.3 ENERGY EXPENDITURE

Within the body, the macronutrients are oxidized by a variety of biochemical pathways, and the energy released in this overall oxidative process is used mainly to synthesize ATP from ADP and inorganic phosphate. The ATP is then utilized to drive biosynthetic reactions, to maintain electrochemical gradients across membranes, and to perform mechanical work via contractile proteins. The efficiency with which ATP synthesis and hydrolysis is coupled to these reactions is not particularly high, so that around 75 per cent of the energy is lost as heat. The total amount of heat produced plus the amount of useful work done is called the energy expenditure.

Energy expenditure can be measured by either direct or indirect calorimetry. Strictly speaking, direct calorimetry measures heat loss rather than heat production, and because of cyclic changes in body temperature these two processes are not always in phase. Thus, direct calorimetry can only be used to assess heat production over periods of at least 24 hours, and since calorimeter chambers are usually rather small this may not be very pleasant for the subject. Hence direct calorimetry is mainly used in the study of temperature regulation.

■ 2.3.1 INDIRECT CALORIMETRY

Indirect calorimetry involves measuring the amounts of oxygen consumed and carbon dioxide produced by respiration. Table 2.4 shows the average amounts of oxygen consumed and carbon dioxide produced per gram of each of the major nutrients, although clearly there will be small differences depending on the exact composition of the substrate, particularly in the case of fats. However, it can be seen that the amount of heat produced per unit oxygen consumed is virtually the same (approximately 20 kJ/l O_2; 4.9 kcal/l O_2) for all substrates. Hence for practical purposes it is sufficient to measure the rate of oxygen consumption in order to calculate energy expenditure.

> Energy expenditure is usually measured by indirect calorimetry. This involves measuring oxygen consumption

The ratio of the amounts of carbon dioxide produced to the amount of oxygen consumed is known as the Respiratory Exchange Ratio (RER, sometimes also called the respiratory quotient), and this varies from 0.7 when pure fat is being oxidized to 1.0 when pure carbohydrate is being oxidized. The amount of amino acids being oxidized can be calculated from measurements of urinary nitrogen excretion, so that when this is combined with measurements of gas exchange it is possible to calculate the amounts of each of the three major nutrients being oxidized (see Box 2.1).

Oxygen consumption can be measured in a number of different ways. The simplest is for the subject to breathe through a mouthpiece into a large bag, called a Douglas bag, for a known period of time, after which the volume of gas exhaled and its oxygen content can be measured. The oxygen content of the inspired air will be that of the atmosphere (20.9 per cent at sea level), so this is sufficient information to calculate oxygen

Table 2.4 Average amounts of oxygen consumed and carbon dioxide produced during the oxidation of metabolic fuels

Nutrient	O_2 consumed (l/g)	CO_2 produced (l/g)	RER (CO_2/O_2)	Energy released (kJ/g)	Energy/O_2 (kJ/l)
Carbohydrate	0.83	0.82	1.0	17.5	21.1
Fat	1.98	1.40	0.71	39.1	19.8
Protein	0.96	0.78	0.81	18.5	19.3
Alcohol	1.43	0.97	0.66	29.8	20.4

■ **BOX 2.1 USE OF DATA FROM INDIRECT CALORIMETRY TO CALCULATE ENERGY EXPENDITURE, RESPIRATORY EXCHANGE RATIO AND THE AMOUNTS OF THE THREE MAJOR NUTRIENTS BEING OXIDIZED**

In one day: oxygen consumption (VO_2) = 600 l

carbon dioxide production (VCO_2) = 525 l

urinary nitrogen excretion (N_U) = 11 g

It is assumed that no alcohol is being metabolized;

Then respiratory exchange ratio = VO_2/VCO_2

$$= 525/600$$

$$= 0.875$$

Energy expenditure, using the formula of Brockway (1987):

$$EE = 16.58\ VO_2 + 4.51\ VCO_2 - 5.90\ N_U\ kJ$$

$$= 16.58 \times 600 + 4.51 \times 525 - 5.90 \times 11.0\ kJ$$

$$= 9948 + 2368 - 65\ kJ$$

$$= 12251\ kJ$$

Carbohydrate oxidation, using the formula of McNeill (2000)

$$= 4.707\ VCO_2 - 3.340\ VO_2 - 2.714\ N_U\ g$$

$$= 4.707 \times 525 - 3.340 \times 600 - 2.714 \times 11\ g$$

$$= 2471 - 2004 - 30\ g$$

$$= 437\ g$$

Fat oxidation, using the formula of McNeill (2000)

$$= 1.786\ VO_2 - 1.778\ VCO_2 - 2.021\ N_U\ g$$

$$= 1.786 \times 600 - 1.778 \times 525 - 2.021 \times 11\ g$$

$$= 1072 - 933 - 22\ g$$

$$= 113\ g$$

---

consumption and hence energy expenditure. The most widely used formula for this purpose is known as the Weir formula

$$\text{energy expenditure (kJ/min)} = V(4.376 - 0.209 \cdot O_E)$$

where V is the volume of breath exhaled per minute, reduced to standard temperature and pressure, and O_E is the percentage oxygen content of the expired gas (see Box 2.2 for a worked example).

■ **BOX 2.2 CALCULATION OF ENERGY EXPENDITURE WHILE STANDING FROM MEASUREMENTS OF OXYGEN CONSUMPTION ALONE, USING A DOUGLAS BAG**

The subject breathed into the Douglas bag for exactly 7 minutes. The volume of gas collected was 73.9 l, and its oxygen content was 17.4 per cent. The temperature of the gas was 23 °C, and atmospheric pressure was 688 mm Hg.

The gas volume is first reduced to STP, using a factor derived from standard tables for air saturated with water vapour. For this temperature and pressure the factor is 0.8092, so the volume at STP is 73.9 × 0.8092 = 59.8 l.

Dividing by 7 minutes,

$$V = 59.8 / 7$$

$$= 8.54 \text{ l/min}$$

$$O_E = 17.4$$

Using the formula of Weir (1949):

$$\text{Energy expenditure} = V \times (4.376 - 0.209 \times O_E)$$

$$= 8.54 \times (4.376 - 0.209 \times 17.4)$$

$$= 8.54 \times (4.376 - 3.637)$$

$$= 8.54 \times 0.739$$

$$= 6.31 \text{ kJ/min (1.51 kcal/min)}$$

A full Douglas bag is rather cumbersome to carry around, and even a 100 l bag fills quite rapidly during any form of exercise, so more portable apparatus has been developed for measuring energy expenditure during non-sedentary activities. Examples are the Kofranyi-Michaelis respirometer, which monitors expired volume continuously and collects a small sample of the expired gas; and the Oxylog, which monitors both expired volume and oxygen content of expired gas continuously. These techniques have allowed the energy costs of a wide range of activities to be determined (see Table 2.5). Such

Table 2.5 Representative values for energy expenditure during a range of activities (values are expressed as multiples of basal metabolic rate)

Activity	Multiple of BMR
Sitting	1.2
Standing	1.4
Walking	3.2
Walking up stairs	6
Running	8
Office work	1.5
Labouring	4

values can then be used in combination with a diary recording the activities performed, say every five minutes, to estimate a person's energy expenditure over a whole day.

Experimental subjects may find the use of a mouthpiece (or a mask) uncomfortable, and may prefer a ventilated hood. This involves placing the subject's head inside a hood, box or small tent attached to a pump which draws room air at a known rate past the subject's face and then through the sensors of oxygen and carbon dioxide analysers. This technique can only be used if the subject remains in one place. Nevertheless, it is currently the method of choice for clinical investigations and short-term metabolic studies.

■ BOX 2.3 CALCULATION OF ENERGY EXPENDITURE USING DOUBLY LABELLED WATER

The subjects consume a single dose of $^2H_2{}^{18}O$, and urine samples are collected over the next 20 days. The isotopic enrichment of urinary water is measured by isotope ratio mass spectrometry.

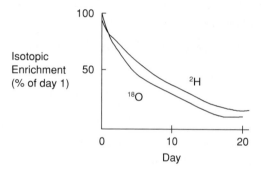

From these graphs' rate constants are calculated for the rate of change of enrichment of oxygen (k_O) and hydrogen (k_D). Then the rate of production of CO_2 (R_{CO_2}) is given by:

$$R_{CO_2} = 0.5N(k_O - k_D)$$

where N is the total body water content.

Typical values are N = 2000 mol, k_O = 0.110/d, k_D = 0.088/d

Thus R_{CO_2} = 0.5 × 2000 × (0.110 − 0.088) = 22 mol/d

To convert this to a value for energy expenditure requires information on the respiratory exchange ratio. It is usually assumed that this can be calculated from the amounts of protein, fat and carbohydrate consumed during the experimental period. A typical value for respiratory exchange ratio on a mixed diet would be 0.85. This corresponds to a value of 23.9 kJ per litre of CO_2 produced, or 534 kJ per mole.

Thus energy expenditure = 22 × 534 = 11760 kJ/d

Note: this is a very simplified version of the calculation – there are a number of other correction factors that have to be applied in practice.

For longer-lasting metabolic studies, where the subject needs to be able to carry out normal daily activities, calorimeters the size of a whole room have been constructed. Again the principle is simply to draw air through the room and to monitor continuously the oxygen and carbon dioxide content of the air that leaves the room. A subject can stay in the room for several days, receiving known amounts of food. This allows extremely accurate balances of fat, carbohydrate and protein, as well as energy, to be calculated.

Confining an experimental subject to a single room for several days does not allow the true energy expenditure of free-living people to be measured. One method which has recently been developed in an attempt to achieve that objective is known as the doubly labelled water method. This requires the subjects to ingest a single dose of water which has been labelled with two stable (i.e. non-radioactive) isotopes, deuterium (^{2}H) and ^{18}O. Samples of a body fluid (usually either saliva or urine) are then collected at intervals over several days, the enrichment of both isotopes is measured and their rate of change with time is calculated, in both cases as complex curvilinear functions. The rate of loss of ^{2}H depends on the rate at which water is being lost, while the rate of loss of ^{18}O depends on the rate of loss of water and carbon dioxide, so that the difference between the two disappearance rates allows the rate of carbon dioxide production to be calculated. This in turn allows energy expenditure to be calculated if the proportions of the different fuels being oxidized is known, and this is usually assumed to be the same as the composition of the diet.

■ 2.3.2 COMPONENTS OF ENERGY EXPENDITURE

It is convenient to consider energy expenditure as consisting of a basal component plus various increments related to physical activity, eating, keeping warm and the response to drugs and hormones. The heat produced by these incremental components is sometimes known as thermogenesis.

The basal metabolic rate is defined as the energy expenditure of a person lying down at complete physical and mental rest in a thermoneutral environment at least twelve hours after eating, drinking or smoking. This can be difficult to achieve in practice, and most experimental determinations are more correctly known as the resting metabolic rate. This is a measure of the energy required for normal metabolic reactions, including the turnover of protein and RNA, the maintenance of cellular sodium and potassium gradients, muscle and vascular tone, breathing, heartbeat, etc.

The major determinants of basal metabolic rate are body size and composition. Adipose tissue has a much lower metabolic rate per unit mass than lean tissue, and this is largely because so much of the adipose tissue mass consists of relatively inert deposits of triacylglycerol. Age and sex also affect basal metabolic rate. This is mainly due to their effects on body size and composition, although in children there is also a component associated with the energy cost of growth. There also appears to be a genetic component, since there are reports of differences in metabolic rate of up to 10 per cent between individuals of apparently similar body size and composition, but no genes have yet been identified which account for a consistent or significant proportion of this variation. On the other hand, there is no shortage of suggestions for possible mechanisms leading to different metabolic rates, including differences in the rate of protein turnover, the efficiency of Na:K ATPase, or the activity of various futile metabolic cycles.

Figure 2.1 Components of daily energy expenditure in an 80 kg young male

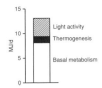

The increment due to physical activity includes both the work done and the heat produced by muscular contraction. It can account for 20–40 per cent of daily energy expenditure. Clearly it varies with the intensity of the exercise or work, but it is also affected by the person's body weight whenever the activity involves moving that weight.

The ingestion of food causes a temporary increase in metabolic rate which may amount to about 10 per cent of the energy content of the meal. This is caused by a variety of processes, including the activity involved in eating and the energy costs of digesting, absorbing and transporting the nutrients and the associated changes in blood flow. However, the major component is the energy utilized in synthesizing and storing glycogen, triacylglycerol and protein. The size of this increment is affected by the composition of the meal, with protein intake causing a slightly greater increase than either fat or carbohydrate intake. For this reason the increment used to be known as the specific dynamic action of protein, although it is now given the more general name of the thermic effect of food or the heat increment of feeding.

Some energy may need to be expended to maintain normal body temperature. Quite a lot of heat is generated inevitably as a by-product of normal metabolic processes, as has been mentioned, but if more heat is needed it can be generated by either non-shivering or shivering thermogenesis. Non-shivering thermogenesis may involve a degree of uncoupling of electron transport from ADP phosphorylation under the influence of a mitochondrial protein named thermogenin. This is an important process in small mammals and human infants, where it occurs particularly in brown adipose tissue. It occurs to a lesser extent in adult human beings, where it tends to be mainly associated with skeletal muscle. Keeping cool by sweating also involves a small increase in energy expenditure.

Many common pharmacological agents cause energy expenditure to rise, including alcohol, nicotine, theophylline and caffeine. Thyroid hormone causes an increase in metabolic rate, as do catecholamines, which may mediate the acute effects of psychological stress on energy expenditure. Cytokines such as tumour necrosis factor and the interleukins may have a similar effect, and thus be responsible for the increase in metabolic rate which occurs in response to infectious, traumatic and inflammatory illnesses.

■ 2.4 ENERGY REQUIREMENTS

An adult person needs to consume just enough food energy to balance their energy expenditure and thus maintain energy balance, hence recommendations for energy intake are based on estimates of energy expenditure. It is clearly impractical to measure every individual's energy expenditure, but there are sufficient data in the literature to allow the development of equations which predict the average energy expenditure of groups of people.

The current recommendations of the authorities in the UK, and indeed the international recommendations of the United Nations Organisation are based on the work of Schofield *et al.* This involves firstly the prediction of basal metabolic rate from body weight, age and sex, using the equations listed in Table 2.6. The result is then multiplied by a ratio known as the physical activity level. This ratio varies from 1.4 to 1.9, depending on the amount of energy likely to be expended in occupational and recreational activities (see Table 2.7). For children, the recommendations also take into account the additional energy costs of growth. For pregnant and lactating women, additional amounts of energy are recommended to allow for the growth of the foetus and the synthesis and

Energy requirements can be estimated from predicted energy expenditure

Table 2.6 Equations for predicting basal metabolic rate (BMR) from body weight (W) measured in kg

	BMR (MJ/d)
Males	10 – 17y BMR = 0.074W + 2.754
	18 – 29y BMR = 0.063W + 2.896
	30 – 59y BMR = 0.048W + 3.653
Females	10 – 17y BMR = 0.056W + 2.898
	18 – 29y BMR = 0.062W + 2.036
	30 – 59y BMR = 0.034W + 3.538

Source: Dietary Reference Values for Food Energy and Nutrients for the United Kingdom (2001).

Table 2.7 Physical activity levels for adults

Non-occupational	Occupational activity					
Activity	Light		Moderate		Heavy	
	Male	Female	Male	Female	Male	Female
Non-active	1.4	1.4	1.6	1.5	1.7	1.5
Moderately active	1.5	1.5	1.7	1.6	1.8	1.6
Very active	1.6	1.6	1.8	1.7	1.9	1.7

Note: These represent the ratio of total energy expenditure to basal metabolic rate.
Source: Dietary Reference Values for Food Energy and Nutrients for the United Kingdom (2001).

secretion of breast milk (see Box 2.4), although there is evidence that metabolic adaptations reduce the expected energy costs of these processes.

■ 2.5 ENERGY BALANCE

Energy balance is defined as the difference between energy intake and expenditure. If intake is greater than expenditure balance is said to be positive, and this leads to net deposition of energy, usually in the form of triacylglycerol in adipose tissue. A negative balance means expenditure is greater than intake, and leads to loss of tissue. Children need to be in modestly positive energy balance during periods of growth, but most people maintain a zero balance most of the time. Obese people tend to be in positive balance for a relatively short time (the so-called active phase of obesity), then maintain balance at a new, stable body weight.

The fact that body weight remains relatively stable in many people (varying less than 1 kg over a one year period) suggests that quite powerful mechanisms exist to control either intake or expenditure, or both. On the other hand, an increasing proportion of the population is becoming obese, which suggests that recent changes in lifestyle have perturbed these normal regulatory mechanisms. For such people to lose weight requires them to achieve negative energy balance. It may require very considerable effort to decrease energy intake and/or increase expenditure sufficiently to overcome the control

---

■ **BOX 2.4 EXAMPLE OF CALCULATION OF ESTIMATED AVERAGE ENERGY REQUIREMENT OF A GROUP OF BREAST-FEEDING WOMEN**

Age: 25 years
Weight: 60 kg
Occupational activity: Moderate
Non-occupational activity: Non-active
Basal metabolic rate (from Table 2.6)

$$BMR = 0.062W + 2.036 \text{ MJ/d}$$

$$= 0.062 \times 60 + 2.036 \text{ MJ/d}$$

$$= 3.720 + 2.036 \text{ MJ/d}$$

$$= 5.756 \text{ MJ/d}$$

Physical activity level (from Table 2.7) = 1.5;
Hence total energy expenditure

$$= 5.756 \times 1.5 \text{ MJ/d}$$

$$= 8.63 \text{ MJ/d}$$

Add increment for lactation (from Dietary Reference Values)

$$= 2.0 \text{ MJ/d}$$

Hence estimated average energy requirement

$$= 8.63 + 2.0 \text{ MJ/d}$$

$$= 10.6 \text{ MJ/d}$$

---

mechanisms which normally act to minimize changes in energy balance. This is one reason why obese people tend to regain weight after losing it by dieting.

It is generally accepted that energy balance is regulated mainly by changes in energy intake. Numerous mechanisms have been demonstrated both in humans and animals by which hunger and satiety are affected by metabolites, particularly glucose or amino acids, or hormones in such a way as to tend to regulate energy intake. For example, much interest currently concerns the hormone leptin which is secreted by adipose tissue and acts on the hypothalamus to suppress appetite. Unfortunately, in humans there are also numerous social, psychological and emotional factors which also affect eating behaviour, and these often seem to override the physiological control mechanisms and disturb energy balance. The unprecedented increase in obesity over the past decade has been attributed to an obesogenic environment, where food is in abundance and physical activity is minimized (e.g. the use of cars, computers and watching television).

> ■ **BOX 2.5 CONSEQUENCES OF FAILURE TO CONTROL**
> **ENERGY BALANCE**
>
> The average intake of adult males in the UK is around 10 MJ per day. If energy intake exceeded energy expenditure by just 10 per cent, this would result in a positive energy balance of 1 MJ per day. Over a year this would amount to 365 MJ which would be stored as fat. The energy cost of storing 1 kg fat is about 42 MJ so this would be estimated to lead to an accumulation of 8.7 kg fat, and as body fat contains about 25 per cent water this would lead to a weight gain of about 11.6 kg. However, in practice weight gain is likely to be less than this because more energy has to be expended in carrying around the extra weight. Furthermore, basal metabolic rate increases slightly with increasing energy intake.

Some components of energy expenditure also act to minimize, though not prevent, perturbations in energy balance. Thus postprandial thermogenesis increases with meal size, acting to dissipate some of the excess energy consumed. Any tissue which is laid down increases the overall basal metabolic load of the body, and increases the energetic cost of moving the body.

In small mammals there is good evidence of further adaptive changes in energy expenditure. Thus when rats are over-fed they show a considerable increase in energy expenditure, mediated largely by an increase in non-shivering thermogenesis in brown adipose tissue. This lasts for as long as the overfeeding continues, and in some cases completely prevents additional weight gain. Although there is some evidence for similar adaptive changes in humans, it is far from conclusive.

Attempts to induce a negative energy balance in order to lose weight focus on reducing energy intake. Hundreds of different approaches to dieting have been proposed, many of which work for at least some people. However, they only work if they succeed in decreasing energy intake, since energy from one nutrient or foodstuff is just as fattening as the same amount of energy from any other nutrient or foodstuff. The only difference between different diets is the way in which the energy intake is reduced, and the way in which the desire to overeat is controlled. There are also some drugs which can help to suppress appetite, including amphetamines, fenfluramine and diethylpropion. These all have undesirable side-effects, including addiction in some cases, and most tend to become less effective with repeated use.

Decreased energy expenditure is an important cause of weight gain. However, there is less scope for losing weight by increasing energy expenditure. It is difficult to sustain increased levels of physical activity to an extent that will achieve more than about a 10 per cent increase in energy expenditure. This will not achieve an encouraging rate of weight loss, although it may be useful in maintaining a stable weight after the desired weight loss has been achieved, and it does have a beneficial effect on the cardiovascular system and decreases the risk of developing Type II diabetes (see Chapter 9). There is considerable research activity devoted to finding a drug which will increase metabolic rate, with much of the current focus being on β_3-adrenergic agonists, but so far none has been found which is sufficiently safe and effective.

SUMMARY

- Energy is derived from the oxidation of protein, fat, carbohydrate and alcohol by reactions that are coupled to the synthesis of ATP.
- Metabolizable energy is the amount of energy that is available to the body for ATP synthesis, after correcting for urinary and faecal losses.
- Fat has a metabolizable energy value of 37 kJ/g, carbohydrate 16 kJ/g, protein 17 kJ/g and alcohol 29 kJ/g.
- Energy expenditure is usually measured by indirect calorimetry, which involves measuring oxygen consumption and carbon dioxide production.
- The main components of energy expenditure are basal metabolic rate, thermogenesis and physical activity.
- Energy requirements are derived from measurements of energy expenditure needed to maintain energy balance. Energy requirements for groups of people can be predicted from their age, weight, sex and physical activity level.

FURTHER READING

Brockway, J.M. (1987) 'Derivation of formulae used to calculate energy expenditure in man', *Hum. Nutr. Clin. Nutr*, 41C: 463–71.

Department of Health (1991) *Dietary Reference Values for Food Energy and Nutrients for the United Kingdom*. Report on Health and Social Subjects, 41. London: HMSO.

Girardier, L. and Stock, M.J. (1983) *Mammalian thermogenesis*. London: Chapman and Hall.

James, W.P.T., Schofield, C. and Schofield, W.N. (1985) 'Basal metabolic rate – review and prediction', *Hum. Nutr. Clin. Nutr*, 39 (suppl): 1–96.

McCance and Widdowson's The Composition of Foods, Sixth Summary Edition. (2002) London: Royal Society of Chemistry.

McNeill, G. (1999) *Energy intake and expenditure* in Garrow, J.S., James, W.P.T. and Ralph, A. (eds) *Human Nutrition and Dietetics*. London: Churchill Livingstone.

Saltiel, A.R. (2001) 'You are what you secrete', *Nat Med*, 7(8): 887–8.

Schoeller, D.A. and van Santen, E. (1982) 'Measurement of energy expenditure in humans by doubly labelled water method', *J. Appl. Physiol*, 53: 955–9.

Weir, J.B. de V. (1949) 'New methods for calculating metabolic rate with special reference to protein metabolism', *J. Physiol*, 109: 1–9.

WHO. 'Energy and protein requirements', report of a joint FAO/WHO/UNU Expert Consultation, Geneva, 1985.

PROTEIN

■ 3.1 THE NEED FOR PROTEIN

Protein is a major component of all living cells, and thus of the human body. It makes up about 17 per cent of the weight of an average adult, making it the second biggest component after water. It forms the building blocks of tissues, enzymes and chemical messengers (see Table 3.1). The need for protein during growth is self evident – it is needed to make up new tissue. What is not so obvious is the need for protein in a non-growing adult. A certain amount of tissue protein is broken down to amino acids each day; some of these amino acids are oxidized or irreversibly converted to other compounds. Protein is also lost from the body as dead skin, hair, nails and intestinal secretions. Thus dietary protein is needed to replace that which is lost.

Protein is an inevitable component of any diet based on the consumption of other organisms. Although it is possible to extract purified products containing just fat or just carbohydrate, as soon as one consumes any cellular material there is protein present.

Table 3.1 Functions of proteins within the body

Function	Examples
Catalysis	Enzymes
Storage and transport	Ferritin
	Haemoglobin
	Amino acid transporters
Structure	Collagen
	Elastin
Contraction	Actin
	Myosin
Communication	Hormones
	Receptors

Note: This list is not exhaustive, but illustrates some of the range of functions for which proteins are responsible.

Thus it is very unusual to find a diet that is very low in protein, and it is consumed in adequate amounts by most people.

■ 3.2 PROTEIN CHEMISTRY

Proteins are macromolecules made up of chains of amino acids joined together by peptide bonds. There are 20 different amino acids which can be incorporated into proteins, although some of them can be chemically modified after incorporation, so that hydrolysis of a mature protein can yield in excess of this number.

Amino acids can be represented by a common formula (see Figure 3.1). The R group is different for each different amino acid, and this affects not only the chemical and physical properties of the amino acid but also the structure and function of the protein which contains it (see Table 3.2).

• **Figure 3.1** The common formula for amino acids

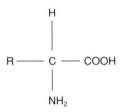

Since different proteins contain different proportions of the different amino acids, their elemental composition will each be slightly different. However, they will all contain carbon, hydrogen, oxygen and nitrogen, and most will also contain sulphur. The most useful feature of this composition from a nutritional point of view is the nitrogen content. This distinguishes protein from the other major components of both tissues and foodstuffs – water, fat and carbohydrate do not contain nitrogen. This means that if we want to measure the protein content of a food, or of a sample of tissue, all we have to do is to measure the nitrogen content. This is very useful because different proteins have such a wide variety of physical and chemical properties that it would be difficult to separate them all and measure them in any other way.

Proteins contain nitrogen as well as carbon, hydrogen and oxygen

The nitrogen content is also important in metabolic terms. Once the protein from food has entered the body it is broken down and metabolized to a variety of other substances, and these are excreted in various different forms, but again the feature which distinguishes them as end products of protein metabolism is the nitrogen content. So for practical reasons we tend to measure nitrogen metabolism, and this becomes synonymous with protein metabolism.

■ 3.2.1 MEASUREMENT OF PROTEIN CONTENT

The protein content of foodstuffs is usually measured by determining the nitrogen content using the Kjeldahl method. This can be used to measure the total nitrogen content of tissue samples, or urine, faeces or other physiological specimens. The method involves digesting the sample for several hours in hot concentrated sulphuric acid. The digestion rate can be increased by the addition of catalysts, and an inert solute to raise the boiling point. The carbon and hydrogen are oxidized to carbon dioxide and water, while the

Nitrogen is measured by the Kjeldahl method which converts amino nitrogen into ammonia

Table 3.2 Structure of amino acids

Common feature	Name	Structure
Aliphatic side chains	Glycine	
	Alanine	
Branched chain amino acids	Leucine	
	Isoleucine	
	Valine	
Aromatic side chains	Tryptophan	
	Tyrosine	
	Phenylalanine	

Table 3.2 *(con't)*

Common feature	Name	Structure
Hydroxy side chains	Serine	
	Threonine	
Sulphur containing amino acids	Cysteine	
	Methionine	
Acids and amides	Glutamic Acid	
	Glutamine	
	Aspartic Acid	
	Asparagine	
Basic side chains	Lysine	

Table 3.2 *(con't)*

Common feature	Name	Structure
	Arginine	
	Histidine	
Imino acids	Proline	

nitrogen is reduced to ammonia. The amount of ammonia produced can then be measured by a variety of colorimetric or titrimetric methods.

The measured nitrogen content is then converted to a protein content on the basis that the average nitrogen content of protein is 16 per cent. Most people find it easier to multiply than to divide, so instead of dividing by 0.16, nitrogen content is multiplied by 6.25 to give protein content.

There are three limitations to this method for determining the protein content of a food:

1   It measures all the nitrogen, including that in molecules other than protein. For example, it would include nucleic acids. These make up no more than 1–2 per cent of the nitrogen in most foods, and so can be ignored, but there are exceptions such as mushrooms, in which 60 per cent of the nitrogen is non-protein nitrogen.
2   Not all the nitrogen gets converted to ammonia by the Kjeldahl method. This mainly applies to compounds in which the nitrogen is bonded to oxygen (which doesn't include the nitrogen in protein). In any case, it is only a very small proportion of the nitrogen in foodstuffs, and can safely be ignored.
3   Not all proteins contain exactly 16 per cent N. For example, cereals contain rather more, so for wheat flour the figure is N × 5.70. On the other hand milk contains rather less, so for milk and milk products the figure is N × 6.38.

The value obtained from Kjeldahl N × 6.25 is referred to as the **crude protein** content of the food. This term does not imply any imprecision or inaccuracy in the measurement – indeed it is a very precise definition – but it simply recognizes that it is not a true measure of the protein content. However, other biochemical methods for measuring protein content such as those based on the biuret reaction tend not to be appropriate for most foodstuffs, where it may be difficult to extract the protein quantitatively from a complex matrix and where the proportions of different amino acids may vary widely between the different food proteins.

Crude protein =
N × 6.25

■ 3.3 FOOD SOURCES

Virtually all the food we consume, both plant and animal, contains some protein. Some foods are considered as 'protein foods', which means that they contain a relatively high concentration of protein. The main examples are meat, fish, milk, cheese, eggs and legumes, especially soya beans. However, the importance of any food as a source of any nutrient also depends on the amount of that food that is eaten, so foods that we eat a lot of are important sources of many nutrients.

On a worldwide basis by far the most important sources of protein are cereals. It is worth noting that, for a diet based on cereals, if people are able to consume enough to satisfy their energy needs they will also have consumed enough to satisfy their protein needs. This does not apply to diets based on starchy roots such as cassava and plantains, which have a much lower ratio of protein to energy, so that people need to eat significant quantities of other protein sources such as beans, cereals or animal products as well.

Cereals are major
sources of protein in
human diets

The major sources of protein in the diets of women following an omnivorous or vegetarian diet living in the UK are shown in Figure 3.2.

Note that meat is the biggest source of protein in the average diet in the UK, in common with other developed countries. Protein intakes are lower in vegetarians but a higher contribution is derived from cereals and other plant-based foods. In vegan diets, cereals and pulses both provide about one-third of the intake. However, the total protein intake of vegans and vegetarians is only slightly lower than that of omnivores.

Adults in this country eat on average 73 g protein per day (men 85 g, women 62 g). However, the most useful way to look at quantity is as a proportion of energy, to take account of differences in total food intake. In almost all diets around the world this proportion is between 10 and 15 per cent, with relatively small differences between poorer

• **Figure 3.2** Sources of dietary protein in omnivore and vegetarian women in the UK (*Source*: Adapted from Reddy S and Sanders TAB, 1990)

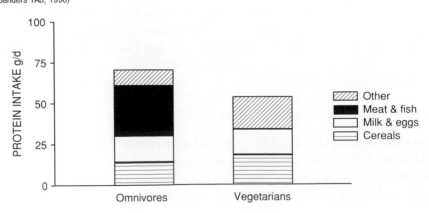

countries and richer ones. In the UK the average protein intake in men is 14.1 per cent of energy, while for women it is 15.2 per cent. The proportion increases slightly with age, as energy intake falls. It has also been increasing slightly over recent years, again as energy intake has fallen. Finally, there is a small social class gradient in the UK, from approximately 14.7 per cent in the highest social class A to 14.3 per cent in social class D.

Human diets contain a huge variety of different proteins, but from a nutritional point of view differences in their biochemical functions are not particularly important. Of much greater importance is the proportions of the various amino acids which they contain, and the digestibility of the protein within the human gut. These two properties determine the **quality** of the protein (see below), which must be considered when evaluating whether a given quantity of protein will satisfy nutritional needs.

■ 3.4 DIGESTION, ABSORPTION AND METABOLISM

The classical view is that proteins are hydrolysed in the stomach and small intestine to amino acids, which are then absorbed from the small intestine. These free amino acids then circulate in the bloodstream to all the organs and tissues of the body, where they are metabolized. This is a reasonable description of the overall process, although it is now clear that the uptake of small peptides, 2–5 amino acids long, is also quite important.

Proteins are digested in the gut and enter the circulation as a mixture of free amino acids

■ 3.4.1 DIGESTION

The stomach secretes a series of enzymes which are collectively known as pepsins. These enzymes have different pH optima ranging from just below neutral, corresponding to the conditions within the stomach immediately after a meal, to pH 1.2, as would be found there several hours later. They begin the process of breaking the proteins up into smaller peptides by hydrolysing peptide bonds adjacent to phenylalanine, tyrosine and leucine residues.

Most protein digestion occurs in the small intestine by the action of enzymes which are secreted by the exocrine pancreas. Table 3.3 shows the specific sites of secretion of each of these enzymes.

Table 3.3 Digestive proteolytic enzymes

Enzyme	Zymogen
Stomach	
Pepsin	Pepsinogen
Pancreas	
Trypsin	Trypsinogen
Chymotrypsins	Chymotrypsinogens
Elastase	Proelastase
Carboxypeptidases	Procarboxypeptidases
Small intestine	
Enterokinase	–
Aminopeptidases	–

These enzymes are synthesized as inactive proenzymes, or zymogens, in order to avoid them hydrolysing the proteins of the cells in which they are synthesized. They are activated only after being secreted into the duodenum. This activation involves cleaving off a terminal peptide which prevents the normal folding of the mature polypeptide chain. Thus pepsinogen is activated by hydrochloric acid in the stomach. Trypsinogen is activated by enteropeptidase (enterokinase), an enzyme secreted by the small intestine. Trypsin then activates all the other proteolytic enzymes.

There are several factors such as the tertiary structure of the protein and the degree of cross-linking of the peptide chains which can affect the rate of digestion of proteins. Indigestible cell walls may physically hinder the access of digestive enzymes to some plant proteins. Antinutrients such as tannins and trypsin inhibitors (found in raw beans) can inhibit protein digestion either by binding to the digestive enzymes or by forming insoluble complexes with the protein substrate. This results in reduced protein digestibility as well as abdominal discomfort if consumed in large quantities. Digestibility can often be improved by cooking, particularly extended boiling in water which denatures trypsin inhibitors and leaches out tannins. The foodstuffs which most commonly display low digestibility are the legumes, including soya beans.

■ 3.4.2 ABSORPTION

The products of digestion by the pancreatic enzymes are mainly small peptides. The final stage of digestion to free amino acids is carried out by aminopeptidases in the cells lining the small intestine (enterocytes). This hydrolysis may occur just before the amino acids are transported into the cell, or it may occur within the cell. Experiments *in vitro* have indicated that small peptides may actually be transported into these cells rather faster than free amino acids.

Amino acids and small peptides can enter the enterocyte both by passive diffusion and by active transport. The specificities and mechanisms of the amino acid transport systems in the gut appear to be broadly similar to those of the systems which are found in other tissues, particularly the brush border of the kidney tubule (see Table 3.4). The amino acids may then be metabolized within the cell, but the majority diffuse down a concentration gradient into the portal circulation.

■ 3.4.3 METABOLISM

The amino acids which are derived from dietary protein mix with the pool of free amino acids within the body, and can be considered as having three possible metabolic fates. They can be used for protein synthesis, they can be oxidized to urea, carbon dioxide and water, or they can be converted to a variety of other small molecules (see Figure 3.3).

3.4.3.1 Protein synthesis

Even in the non-growing adult there is always some protein being synthesized from amino acids, and this is matched by an equivalent amount of protein being broken down to amino acids. This phenomenon of protein turnover can be demonstrated by feeding isotopically labelled amino acid and observing that a significant proportion of the label is retained in body proteins even though the amount of nitrogen going in as food protein is closely matched by the amount of nitrogen excreted as urea.

Protein turnover means the continual breakdown and resynthesis of tissue proteins

Table 3.4 Intestinal amino acid transport systems

System	Sodium dependence	Preferred amino acids
A	yes	alanine, serine, glycine, methionine, proline
L	no	leucine, isoleucine, valine, methionine, phenylalanine, tyrosine, tryptophan, histidine
ASCP	yes	alanine, serine, cysteine, proline
Ly	yes	lysine, histidine, arginine, ornithine
x_A^-	yes	aspartate
x_G^-	yes	glutamate
x_C^-	no	aspartate, glutamate, cysteine
y^+	yes	lysine, arginine, histidine
β	yes	β-alanine, taurine
$b^{0,+}$	no	lysine, leucine
Gly	yes	glycine, sarcosine
N	yes	histidine, glutamine, asparagine
imino	yes	proline

• **Figure 3.3** Metabolic fates of ingested protein

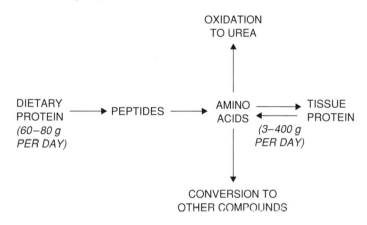

The difference between the rates of protein synthesis and breakdown determines whether the mass of protein in the body increases, for instance during growth, or decreases, for instance during wasting diseases. Nutrient intake is one factor which can affect rates of protein synthesis and breakdown, with both tending to decrease if protein or energy intakes are inadequate. However, protein turnover does continue even if intake is zero. In this case an obligatory level of protein breakdown occurs, releasing amino acids of which a proportion can be recycled to maintain protein synthesis.

Protein synthesis is quantitatively the biggest process for disposal of amino acids. It has been shown that an adult synthesizes 3–400 g protein each day, even though intake may be only 60–80 g per day. The rates of protein synthesis and breakdown are always very close. Even the most rapidly growing young infant would only be depositing protein at a net rate of approximately 10 g per day, while he or she is turning over 50–100 g protein per day.

3.4.3.2 Oxidation

Ultimately, all the amino acids that enter the body will be disposed of by oxidation. Some will be retained as tissue protein for a time, but this is matched by an equal amount of amino acids being released from tissue protein to be oxidized.

The amino acid can be considered in two parts, as a carbon skeleton and an amino group. The amino group is oxidized to urea in the liver; the urea then circulates to the kidney, where it is excreted. In fact the rate of urea production is somewhat greater than the rate of urea excretion in the urine: the difference is called urea salvage. This occurs in the large intestine where urea can be hydrolysed to ammonia by bacteria. This ammonia diffuses back into the circulation, and can be reutilized for the synthesis of non-essential amino acids.

The carbon skeleton of the amino acid is oxidized to carbon dioxide and water, with the release of energy as ATP. Thus amino acids form one of the major fuel sources for the liver, in particular. Moreover one particular amino acid, glutamine, is the major fuel for the gut and for white blood cells.

Under certain circumstances, such as starvation, diabetes or a high fat diet, the body may need to synthesize glucose from amino acids rather than oxidizing them directly. Experiments with diabetic dogs fed on single amino acids have shown that most of the amino acids can be converted to glucose, and are therefore classified as **glucogenic**. However, leucine and lysine cannot be converted to glucose, and under these circumstances they give rise to acetoacetic acid, so they are classified as **ketogenic**. This classification can be related to the pathways by which the amino acids are catabolized. The ketogenic amino acids are those that are metabolized only to acetyl CoA, while those that are metabolized to TCA cycle intermediates are glucogenic. Tryptophan, methionine and cysteine produce pyruvate and so can be either ketogenic or glucogenic. Phenylalanine and tyrosine are metabolized to fumarate plus acetoacetate and are thus both ketogenic and glucogenic, as is isoleucine, which is metabolized to acetyl CoA plus succinyl CoA.

3.4.3.3 Other metabolic pathways

The third possibility is that some amino acids can be metabolized to other molecules such as hormones and nucleic acids, including those shown in Table 3.5.

Some amino acids will also be converted to other amino acids in order to supply the appropriate balance of substrates for protein synthesis. Again, the amino group and the

Table 3.5 Examples of other molecules to which amino acids may be converted

Amino acid	Product
Arginine	Creatine, NO
Aspartate	Nucleic acid bases
Glutamine	Nucleic acid bases
Glycine	Creatine, haem, bile acids
Lysine	Carnitine
Methionine	Creatine
Tryptophan	5-hydroxytryptamine, nicotinic acid
Tyrosine	Catecholamines, thyroid hormones, melanin

Amino acids are catabolized to urea, carbon dioxide and water, with the release of energy

carbon skeleton must be considered separately. The amino group can be transferred from almost any amino acid to almost any other by the action of transaminase enzymes. The only amino acids which don't appear to participate in transamination reactions are lysine and threonine.

The situation with the carbon skeletons is more complicated. There are some amino acids whose carbon skeletons can be made from other amino acids, or indeed from other metabolic intermediates which may be derived from carbohydrate or fat. These are known as **non-essential** or dispensable amino acids. Amino acids whose carbon skeletons cannot be made from other dietary constituents are known as **essential** or indispensable amino acids, and these must be supplied in adequate quantities by the diet.

Essential amino acids are those whose carbon skeletons cannot be synthesized in the human body

■ 3.5 CLASSIFICATION OF AMINO ACIDS AS ESSENTIAL OR NON-ESSENTIAL

This concept arose originally from a series of classic nutritional experiments by W.C. Rose in the 1930s. In the first series he fed young, rapidly growing rats on purified diets containing adequate amounts of fat, carbohydrate, vitamins and minerals together with mixtures of all the 20 amino acids which were known to be present in proteins. He then removed one amino acid at a time from the diet. Two types of response were observed. For some amino acids the removal made no difference – the rats continued to grow at the same rate. These amino acids could thus be described as non-essential (see Table 3.6). For others the response was dramatic – the rats stopped growing, then lost weight, lost appetite, and eventually died. These amino acids were described as essential. The result of removing arginine was somewhat ambiguous, as the rats still grew but at a much reduced rate.

Further experiments showed that rats could synthesize the non-essential amino acids themselves, however they could not synthesize the essential amino acids, so that when one of these was excluded from the diet they could not synthesize any protein, since

Table 3.6 Essential and non-essential amino acids for the rat and humans

Essential		Non-essential	
Rat	*Man*	*Rat*	*Man*
Leucine	Leucine	Tyrosine*	Tyrosine*
Valine	Valine	Cysteine†	Cysteine†
Threonine	Threonine	Aspartic acid	Aspartic acid
Methionine	Methionine	Asparagine	Asparagine
Phenylalanine	Phenylalanine	Glumatic acid	Glumatic acid
Lysine	Lysine	Glutamine	Glutamine
Histidine		Alanine	Alanine
Arginine		Proline	Proline
		Glycine	Glycine
		Serine	Serine
			Histidine
			Arginine

Notes:
*can be synthesized from phenylalanine
†can be synthesized from methionine

virtually all tissue proteins have to contain some of each amino acid. Protein breakdown and amino acid oxidation continued, leading to a continual loss of tissue protein. The rats were able to synthesize arginine, but at a limited rate which was clearly not sufficient to allow optimum growth.

Rose went on to do similar feeding experiments in human volunteers, and found that the two species had slightly different nutritional needs. In these studies he used the **nitrogen balance** technique rather than the growth response as the criterion for adequacy of the diets. This means that he measured the intake and excretion of nitrogen over a period of several days. For an adult on an adequate diet one would expect intake and excretion to be equal. If intake is greater than excretion (positive balance) tissue protein must be being deposited, as occurs during growth. On the other hand if excretion is greater than intake (negative balance) this means that there is a net loss of tissue protein, and indicates that the diet is inadequate.

Rose started with a mixture of the ten essential amino acids from his work on the rats. The volunteers maintained nitrogen balance on this, showing clearly that the other ten amino acids were also non-essential for humans. He then removed each in turn. Removing histidine or arginine made no difference – nitrogen balance was maintained, showing that histidine and arginine are non-essential for humans. But for each of the other amino acids, the volunteers immediately went into sustained negative nitrogen balance as soon as it was removed from their diet. Interestingly, they also complained of symptoms such as fatigue, irritability and loss of appetite. It should be noted that cysteine can only be synthesized from methionine, so the requirements for these two amino acids are normally considered together. The same applies to tyrosine, which can only be synthesized from phenylalanine. Hence cysteine and tyrosine are sometimes referred to as semi-essential amino acids.

Recent work has suggested that there are some conditions involving rapid growth or the recovery from certain illnesses in which the body's capacity to synthesize arginine, histidine, glycine or glutamine can be inadequate, and nitrogen balance can improve when one or other of these amino acids is given in the diet. Thus these amino acids are sometimes classified as conditionally essential.

■ 3.6 PROTEIN QUALITY

Protein quality means the efficiency with which dietary protein is utilized within the body

Protein quality may be defined as the efficiency with which a dietary protein can be utilized by the body. It has two main components: digestibility (i.e. the proportion of ingested protein that is actually absorbed from the gut), and essential amino acid composition relative to requirement.

The best way to understand protein quality is to see how it is measured. There are two main approaches – the so-called biological and chemical methods.

■ 3.6.1 BIOLOGICAL METHODS FOR ASSESSING PROTEIN QUALITY

These involve feeding a group of people or animals on a diet containing a set amount of the test protein for a period of days and measuring an appropriate biological response. The most useful method is called **Net Protein Utilization** (**NPU**). This is defined as the increase in nitrogen retention per unit increase in nitrogen intake, and is commonly abbreviated to

$$NPU = \text{nitrogen retained/nitrogen intake}$$

Outlines of the methods for measuring NPU using experimental animals or human volunteers are given in Boxes 3.1 and 3.2.

■ **BOX 3.1 MEASUREMENT OF NET PROTEIN UTILIZATION (NPU) USING EXPERIMENTAL ANIMALS**

To measure NPU, two diets are formulated with the test protein as the sole source of protein; only the concentration of protein differs between the two diets. The diets are then fed to matched groups of experimental animals, usually rats. Nitrogen retention can be determined as the difference in carcass nitrogen content between the beginning and the end of the test period:

$$N \text{ retention} = B - B_0$$

where B_0 and B are the body nitrogen contents of the rats at the beginning and end of the test period respectively. Hence the difference in nitrogen retention attributable to the two diets

$$= (B_X - B_0) - (B_Y - B_0)$$

$$= B_X - B_Y$$

where B_X and B_Y are the final body nitrogen contents of rats fed on diets X and Y. NPU is defined as the difference in nitrogen retention divided by the difference in nitrogen intake on the two diets:

$$NPU = (B_X - B_Y)/(I_X - I_Y)$$

where I_X and I_Y are the intakes of protein on diets X and Y.
The levels of protein usually chosen for X and Y are 0 and 10 per cent respectively.

The two main components of protein quality, digestibility and essential amino acid composition, can be measured separately. **Digestibility** is defined as the amount absorbed expressed as a proportion of intake, a definition which applies to any nutrient. The amount absorbed can be calculated by subtracting the amount excreted in the faeces from the amount consumed, i.e.:

$$N \text{ digestibility} = N \text{ absorbed/N intake}$$

$$= (I - F)/I$$

where I is nitrogen intake and F is faecal nitrogen. This is actually the definition of apparent digestibility, and needs be corrected for endogenous losses – intestinal secretions, bacterial cells and intestinal mucosal cells which are sloughed off by the passage of digesta:

$$\text{True N digestibility} = \frac{(I - I_k) - (F - F_k)}{(I - I_k)}$$

where I_k and F_k are the intake and faecal excretion of nitrogen on a protein-free diet. This formula simplifies to:

$$\text{True N digestibility} = \frac{I - (F - F_k)}{I}$$

True digestibility is apparent digestibility corrected for endogenous losses

so long as I_k is zero.

If NPU is now divided by digestibility we get a quantity which is known as the **biological value** (BV). This is defined as the increase in nitrogen retention per unit increase in nitrogen absorbed. It is generally assumed to be mainly a reflection of how well the pattern of amino acids absorbed from the gut matches the requirement for tissue deposition.

■ **BOX 3.2 MEASUREMENT OF NET PROTEIN UTILIZATION USING HUMAN VOLUNTEERS**

It is possible to calculate nitrogen retention from measurements of intake and excretion during a balance period of five days on a diet containing the test protein as sole nitrogen source. The major routes of nitrogen excretion are urine and faeces, so that

$$\text{nitrogen retention} = I - U - F$$

where I is nitrogen intake and U and F are urinary and faecal nitrogen excretion respectively. NPU is defined as the difference in nitrogen retention divided by the difference in nitrogen intake:

$$\text{NPU} = (I_X - U_X - F_X) - (I_Y - U_Y - F_Y)/(I_X - I_Y)$$

where the subscripts refer to intake and excretion on two diets X and Y.

■ **3.6.2 CHEMICAL METHODS FOR ASSESSING PROTEIN QUALITY**

In order to avoid the need for numerous biological assays a number of *in vitro* procedures have been developed for predicting aspects of protein quality. Digestibility is usually measured by incubating the test protein with a mixture of proteolytic enzymes, including porcine trypsin, chymotrypsin and intestinal peptidase, and sometimes bacterial proteases. Digestibility can then be determined from the rate at which the pH falls, and this is usually quantified by measuring the rate at which standard alkali has to be added to keep the pH constant.

The adequacy of the amino acid composition of a protein can be assessed by comparing it with an estimate of essential amino acid requirements. The requirements are based on experiments to determine the amounts of essential amino acids needed by pre-school children to achieve optimal nitrogen retention. The resulting pattern of essential amino acid requirements is known as the reference protein, and the result of comparing the amino acid composition of a dietary protein with the reference protein is known as the **amino acid score**.

$$\text{Amino acid score} = \frac{\text{mg amino acid per g test protein} \times 100}{\text{mg amino acid per g reference protein}}$$

Applying this formula to each essential amino acid in turn will produce a series of eight figures. The lowest figure represents the amino acid score of the protein as whole, and generally predicts the biological value quite well.

The amino acid with the lowest score is called the **(first) limiting amino acid**, because it limits the value of the protein. The limiting amino acid is defined as the essential amino acid which is present in the smallest quantity in relation to its requirement, though it is not necessarily the essential amino acid that is present in the lowest absolute amount. Once the limiting amino acid has all been utilized within the body, the remaining amino acid mixture is incomplete, so no more tissue protein can be synthesized.

The limiting amino acid is the essential amino acid that is present in the smallest quantity in relation to its requirement

In practice there are only two or three amino acids that are ever limiting in normal foodstuffs. For cereals it is usually lysine, while for legumes and for most other important protein sources it is methionine. Tryptophan is usually the next limiting amino acid, or occasionally threonine.

In reality, of course, people do not usually consume only a single source of protein. When a whole diet is analysed the amino acid score is rather greater than that of its individual constituents. This is because of the phenomenon of mutual supplementation, whereby a relative shortage of one amino acid in one food is made good by a relative excess of that amino acid in another food. For example, rice is limited by its lysine content while beans are limited by their methionine content. But if they are mixed together, for example in a diet based on rice plus a relish made from beans, there is enough lysine in the beans to make up for what is missing in the rice, and enough methionine in the rice to make up for what is missing in the beans.

For virtually all diets around the world, the amino acid composition is not a limiting factor for adults or older children, but for younger children it can be a significant consideration in some cases, because of their relatively higher requirements for essential amino acids for growth. On the other hand, protein digestibility is a significant factor for many diets around the world. Many vegetable protein sources, particularly legumes and wholegrain cereals, which are the major sources of protein on a worldwide basis, have quite low protein digestibilities. They are very low if they are uncooked, because of antinutrients, but even when they are cooked they may be only 70–80 per cent digestible.

In normal mixed diets protein quality is mainly determined by digestibility

■ 3.7 PROTEIN REQUIREMENTS AND RECOMMENDED INTAKES

The protein intake of an adult is judged to be adequate if the person is able to maintain nitrogen balance, i.e. if the excretion of nitrogenous compounds from the body is equal to the intake of nitrogen, so that the body is neither gaining nor losing nitrogen. For a child the diet must also allow growth at an optimal rate.

Protein requirements are based on the maintenance of nitrogen balance or optimal growth rates

It should be noted that the measurement of nitrogen balance is not simple, and there is a tendency for intake to be overestimated and for excretion to be underestimated, generally because of incomplete collection from the subject. There are many different routes by which nitrogen is lost from the body; as well as urine and faeces nitrogen is lost in sweat, skin, hair, nails, saliva, menstrual blood and semen, and some of these are quite hard to collect reliably. Moreover, even on a constant diet excretion fluctuates by at least one or two grams of nitrogen per day, so that balance may change between positive and negative from day to day. Thus a period of at least four days is needed to make a reliable estimate of nitrogen balance. Nevertheless, no better way of judging the adequacy of protein intakes has yet been established.

One way of trying to predict protein requirements is to measure the loss of nitrogen in subjects fed on a protein-free diet. This endogenous loss amounts to approximately 57 mg N per kg body weight per day for normal adults, equivalent to 0.36 g protein per kg per day. However when people are fed this amount of high quality protein they go into sustained negative nitrogen balance. This is because urinary and faecal nitrogen excretion increase as dietary protein intake increases, so they are higher on an intake of 0.36 g protein/kg/d than on a protein-free diet. In fact it requires an intake of approximately 0.63 g of good quality protein per kg per day on average to maintain nitrogen balance in adults. Thus after making allowances for individual variation in protein requirements, the recommended intake, which should be enough to cover the requirements of virtually all individuals, is usually taken as 0.75 g of good quality protein per kg per day for adults. This figure has to be adjusted upwards if protein quality is low.

For children, similar considerations apply when predicting maintenance requirements. The increment for growth can be calculated from the average rate at which protein is deposited in the body, but again this leads to a figure which is too low to sustain adequate growth rates when tested experimentally. This may be because growth does not normally occur linearly: there are periods of rapid growth interspersed with periods of little or no growth. Thus tables of recommended protein intakes for children at various ages are based on a few experimental observations with interpolation between these points. For infants under 6 months the recommendations are based on the nitrogen content of breast milk.

From a practical point of view, normal diets supply considerably more protein than is implied by the recommended intakes. For example, the estimated average requirement for energy in a moderately active 74 kg adult male is 10.6 MJ/d, and the recommended intake of protein for this person would be 56 g/d, representing 8.7 per cent of the energy intake. But people in the UK actually consume around 15 per cent of their dietary energy as protein. This proportion has increased from about 12 per cent of the energy in the 1970s, mainly because of a decline in the intake of starchy and cereal-based foods such as bread rather than an increase in the absolute protein intake. The trend has been for a decline in the consumption of fatty meats (beef and lamb) and an increase in lean meat such as poultry. Protein intakes are lower in UK vegetarians and vegans (on average 12 per cent of energy intake) but still adequate to maintain a nitrogen balance. Alcoholics are at risk of having an inadequate intake of protein because they derive such a high proportion of their dietary energy from alcohol which dilutes the contribution made by other nutrients. In fact very few diets around the world supply less than 10 per cent of energy as protein, so protein deficiency is not likely to occur if energy intakes are adequate. The diets of children suffering from protein energy malnutrition are usually found to be lacking in energy and many other nutrients rather than being specifically deficient in protein. There is currently no agreement regarding the upper limits to protein intakes.

SUMMARY

- Proteins are macromolecules that are synthesized from 20 different amino acids.
- The protein content in food is measured by analysing its nitrogen content.
- Dietary protein comes from both plant and animal sources.
- Proteins enter the body as a mixture of amino acids which are then used to synthesize tissue proteins or are oxidized to carbon dioxide, water and urea with the production of energy.
- There are eight essential amino acids that must be supplied in the diet.
- Protein quality is a measure of the efficiency with which dietary protein is utilized.
- Protein is required in amounts that will maintain nitrogen balance in adults and support optimal growth in children.

FURTHER READING

Department of Health (1991) *Dietary Reference Values for Food Energy and Nutrients for the United Kingdom*. London: HMSO.

FAO/WHO/UNU (1991) *Assessment of protein quality*. Rome: FAO.

Millward, D.J. (1999) 'The nutritional value of plant-based diets in relation to human amino acid and protein requirements', *Proc. Nutr. Soc*, 58: 249–60.

Reddy, S. and Sanders, T.A.B. (1990) 'Haematological studies on pre-menopausal Indian and Caucasian vegetarians compared with Caucasian omnivores', *British Journal of Nutrition*, 64(2): 331–8.

Rose, W.C. (1957) 'The amino acid requirements of adult man', *Nutrition Abstracts and Reviews*, 27: 631–47.

Waterlow, J.C. (1984) 'Protein turnover with special reference to man', *Quarterly Journal of Experimental Physiology*, 69: 409–38.

WHO. 'Energy and protein requirements', report of a joint FAO/WHO/UNU Expert Consultation, Geneva, 1985.

CARBOHYDRATE

■ 4.1 INTRODUCTION

Carbohydrates are a diverse group of substances which fall into three main groups: sugars, starch and non-starch polysaccharides (dietary fibre). Apart from lactose they are derived almost exclusively from food of plant origin. Plants use the energy from sunlight to synthesize sugars via the process of photosynthesis. The sugars may then be converted to starch for storage or non-starch polysaccharides which form the major structural components of the plant.

Carbohydrate is a major source of energy in most human diets. When there is insufficient carbohydrate in the diet to meet the body's obligatory requirement for glucose (see p 54) it can be synthesized by the process of gluconeogenesis from amino acids (particularly alanine and glutamine), lactic acid or glycerol, though not from fatty acids or alcohol.

Apart from being absorbed and metabolized within the body, carbohydrates can be fermented by bacteria in the mouth and in the large intestine, and these are areas of considerable nutritional significance. Fermentation of soluble carbohydrates in the mouth produces lactic acid which dissolves the enamel of the teeth, leading to dental caries. In the large intestine, fermentation of carbohydrates which have escaped digestion and absorption in the small intestine results in faecal bulking and the formation of short chain volatile fatty acids and gases such as hydrogen, carbon dioxide and methane. It has been argued that some of the effects of colonic bacteria may influence the risk of diseases of the large bowel, particularly cancer (see Chapter 9). It should be noted that most herbivorous species derive the majority of their energy from bacterial fermentation of non-starch polysaccharides. In some species such as the horse and rabbit, this fermentation is also in the hind-gut, but in many others, including cows and sheep, there is a separate organ called the rumen in which fermentation occurs before the digesta passes into the stomach (abomasum) and the intestines.

Carbohydrates consist of sugars, starch and non-starch polysaccharides (dietary fibre)

Glucose cannot be synthesized from fatty acids in humans

■ 4.2 CLASSIFICATION

Carbohydrates have a general molecular formula $(CH_2O)_n$, although many carbohydrates do not quite fit this formula. The following is a strict chemical definition:

> The polyhydroxyaldehydes, -ketones, -alcohols, acids, their simple derivatives and their polymers having polymeric linkages of the acetal type.

In reality the best way to understand what carbohydrates are is to consider a classification based on their nutritional significance. This is summarized in Table 4.1.

Table 4.1 Classification of dietary carbohydrates

	Component	Examples
Sugars	Monosaccharides	Glucose
		Fructose
	Disaccharides	Sucrose
		Lactose
		Maltose
	Sugar alcohols	Sorbitol
		Lactitol
		Xylitol
		Isomalt
		Maltitol
	Oligosaccharides	Raffinose
		Stachyose
		Fructo-oligosaccharides
		Maltodextrins
Polysaccharides	Starch	Amylose
(complex carbohydrates)		Amylopectin
	Glycogen	
	Non-starch polysaccharides	Cellulose
	(dietary fibre)	Hemicellulose
		Pectin
		Gums
		Lignin

A distinction is sometimes made between simple and complex carbohydrates. This is not very helpful because complex carbohydrates include both starch and non-starch polysaccharides, which have very different physiological and nutritional properties.

■ 4.2.1 MONOSACCHARIDES

These are sugars containing 3–7 carbon atoms. Many phosphorylated derivatives are found within the cell as metabolic intermediates. They can be synthesized from most amino acids though not from fatty acids.

The pentoses (ribose and deoxyribose) are very important as components of nucleic acids, but the amounts supplied in the diet are very small. The only free monosaccharides found in significant quantities in food are the hexose sugars, glucose and fructose (see Figure 4.1).

• **Figure 4.1** Structures of monosaccharides

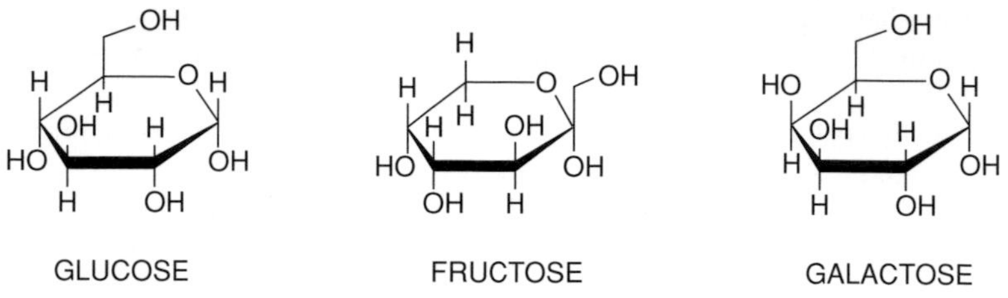

GLUCOSE   FRUCTOSE   GALACTOSE

4.2.1.1 Glucose

Glucose is of central importance because (i) it is the free sugar that is transported in the blood as a fuel for cells and tissues; (ii) it is the basic unit from which glycogen, the storage polysaccharide in animals, is built; and (iii) it is also the basic unit from which starch, the storage polysaccharide in plants is built, and is thus the ultimate product of starch digestion, so it is the form in which most of our dietary carbohydrate enters the circulation. It is also a sub-unit of the structure of the two most common dietary sugars, lactose and sucrose, again adding to the amount of carbohydrate that arrives in the body in this form.

On the other hand, little free glucose is found naturally in foods – some is present in fruits such as grapes and in honey. Athletes often take glucose tablets as a rapid source of energy, although it is certainly absorbed no faster than disaccharides, and only a little faster than starch. Most sports drinks now contain low molecular weight glucose polymers because they release glucose rapidly but have a lower osmolarity than glucose and so promote rehydration.

Glucose is also known as dextrose, particularly in hospitals where it is used in intravenous fluids to maintain blood glucose, for example in shock, and as the main energy source in total parenteral nutrition. In the food industry glucose usually refers to glucose syrups, which are made from partially hydrolysed starch. Pure glucose is again known as dextrose and may be used as a food ingredient or additive since it has useful textural properties and is only about 75 per cent as sweet as sucrose.

4.2.1.2 Fructose

Fructose is the commonest free monosaccharide in the diet, coming mainly from fruit, although much of the sugar in many fruits is actually sucrose. Fructose is also known as laevulose.

Fructose is absorbed relatively slowly from the gut and is metabolized in the liver to glucose derivatives, entering the main glycolytic/gluconeogenic pathway as dihydroxyacetone. It is almost twice as sweet as sucrose, so that less needs to be used to achieve the same sweetening effect. Because of this, as well as its slow absorption and non-insulin dependent metabolism, fructose is used to sweeten specialist diabetic products. However, an excessive intake can lead to diarrhoea caused by the high osmotic pressure it exerts.

In the food industry fructose is usually used in combination with glucose, for example as invert sugar, which is obtained by hydrolysing sucrose to give a 50/50 mixture of glucose and fructose. This mixture does not crystallize, it absorbs water, and is sweeter

• **Figure 4.2** Common dietary disaccharides

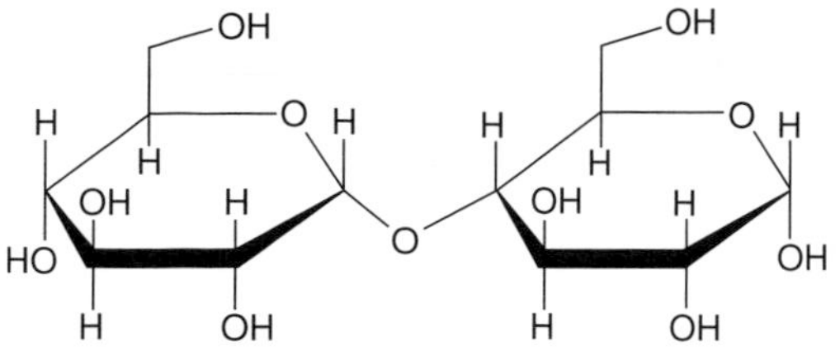

Maltose (glucosyl-glucose)

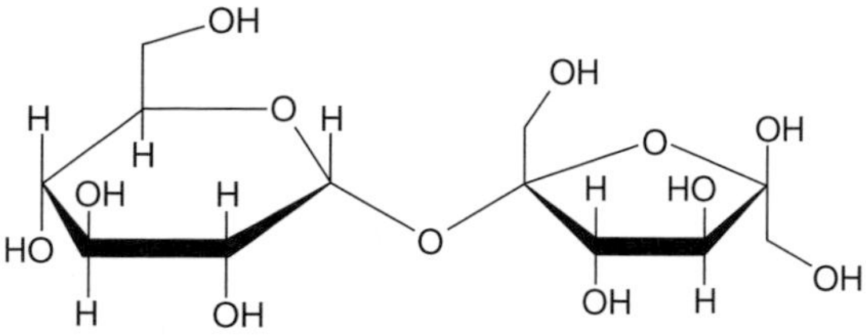

Sucrose (glucosyl-fructose)

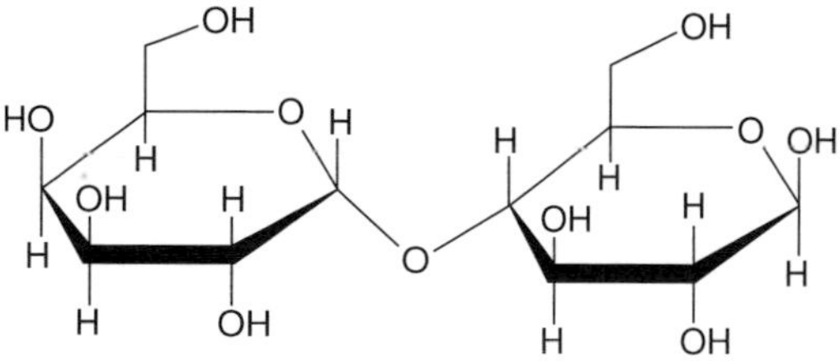

Lactose (galactosyl-glucose)

than sucrose. Alternatively fructose rich syrups can be produced by hydrolysing corn starch to glucose, then inverting about half the glucose to fructose.

■ **4.2.2 DISACCHARIDES**

4.2.2.1 Sucrose

This disaccharide consisting of one glucose and one fructose residue is by far the most common sugar in our diet. Average intake in the UK is around 80 g/day, amounting to around 30 kg in a year. This has declined, however, from a peak of around 50 kg per year in the early 1970s. Less than half is bought as table sugar, with increasing amounts coming from manufactured products and soft drinks.

Sugar has been a major food in the UK only since the latter part of the nineteenth century. It used to be all imported from sugar cane, whereas now most is grown here as beet, making it much cheaper. Sugar consumption tends to rise as countries become more affluent, though it appears never to reach more than 20 per cent of energy intake. Current intakes are around 14 per cent of energy, and it is recommended that this should fall to less than 10 per cent, mainly because of its effects on the teeth.

Table sugar is one of the purest chemicals readily available, being 99.95 per cent sucrose, though even the most unrefined brown sugars contain over 98 per cent sucrose. In this form it is clearly 'empty calories', though it is almost always taken as part of a composite dish which does provide other nutrients.

The main health problem caused by sucrose is dental caries. It is estimated that dental caries becomes prevalent in societies when the intake of sugar exceeds 10 kg per head/year. However, the impact of sugar intake on dental caries is dependent on the presence of dental plaque and the effects are mitigated by exposure to fluoride (see Chapter 9). Moreover, the frequency of intake is probably more important with regard to risk of caries than total intake, though the two are strongly associated.

There is also concern that high sugar diets are more likely to promote overconsumption of energy and hence obesity, though there is little direct evidence to support this. The consumption of sugar-containing carbonated beverages has been associated with the risk of excess weight in childhood when compared with consumption of low-calorie drinks.

Over the years there have also been concerns about the adverse metabolic effects of high sugar consumption, based mainly on animal research, which has shown high concentrations of insulin in the blood, or damage to the liver or kidneys. But the relevance of these findings is questionable as the studies were of diets very high in sugar. There is no evidence that sugar causes diabetes. Furthermore, current dietary advice for diabetics is that it can be consumed in moderation.

> The two most common sugars in the diet are the disccharides sucrose and lactose

4.2.2.2 Lactose

The only other common sugar in our diet is lactose, a disaccharide composed of one glucose and one galactose residue. Average consumption in the UK is estimated to be approximately 15 g/d.

Lactose occurs naturally only in milk, at a concentration of 5 per cent in cow's milk and 7 per cent in human milk. It is present in products made with whole or skimmed milk, but many traditional dairy products exclude the water-soluble fraction. Thus cream contains about half as much lactose as milk, and butter contains virtually none. When cheese is made, some lactose is fermented to lactic acid, and what is left is discarded in the whey fraction. The exception is cottage cheese, which contains a little lactose; there is also some in cheese spreads. Yoghurt also involves fermentation, but only about 25 per cent of the lactose is fermented, and since extra lactose is often added to start the fermentation it may end up with a higher content than whole milk.

Lactose is less sweet than sucrose, and hence is a useful food ingredient, either by itself or with protein in the form of dried skimmed milk. In the newborn, lactose plays an important role in promoting the growth of *Lactobacillus bifidus* in the gut.

4.2.2.3 Maltose

Maltose is a minor component of the diet. It consists of two glucose residues, and occurs mainly as an intermediate of starch digestion. It is found in malted cereal products, having been formed by the partial hydrolysis of starch as the seed grains are allowed to sprout.

■ 4.2.3 OLIGOSACCHARIDES

Sugars containing 3–20 monosaccharide units are known as oligosaccharides. Glucose polymers and maltodextrins are widely used in processed foods. There are a number of non-digestible oligosaccharides (NDO). The most notorious are the trisaccharide raffinose and the tetrasaccharide stachyose, which are found in quite large quantities in legumes (peas and beans), especially soya beans. They are not digested by the enzymes in the mouth or in the small intestine, but can be rapidly fermented by bacteria in the colon, producing the gases carbon dioxide, hydrogen and methane as well as volatile fatty acids. This causes discomfort as well as flatulence, and tends to limit the consumption of legumes by infants and young children who could otherwise benefit from such supplementary protein sources. The content of oligosaccharides can be significantly reduced by soaking and cooking. Inulin is a fructo-oligosaccharide found in Jerusalem artichokes and onions and is responsible for the flatulence which is an effect of eating these foods. Human milk contains NDO in the form of galactooligosaccharides. These are believed to be the *Bifid* factor that promotes the growth of *L. bifidus* in the infant.

■ 4.2.4 POLYSACCHARIDES

4.2.4.1 Starch

Starch makes up more than half the carbohydrate in the diets of even the most affluent countries, and much more in those of poorer countries. Average intakes in the UK are around 130 g/day. The major sources of starch are the traditional staple foods such as cereals, roots and tubers, where it has been deposited in the plant's storage organs.

> Starch is a polymer of glucose and is found in plants

Starch is a mixture of two types of molecule, usually 20–30 per cent amylose and 70–80 per cent amylopectin. Both are made entirely of glucose sub-units. In amylose these are linked by $1–4_\alpha$ bonds in one long straight chain which tends to adopt a helical structure. Amylopectin includes both $1–4_\alpha$ and $1–6_\beta$ links, giving a branched structure (see Figure 4.3). This structure offers more free ends from which amylase enzymes can work, so amylopectin is more rapidly digested.

Raw starch is enclosed in granules which are insoluble and not easily digested. Hence starchy foods need to be cooked before eating. The application of heat and moisture causes the process of gelatinization, by which the granules swell and burst, making the starch

• **Figure 4.3** Structure of amylopectin

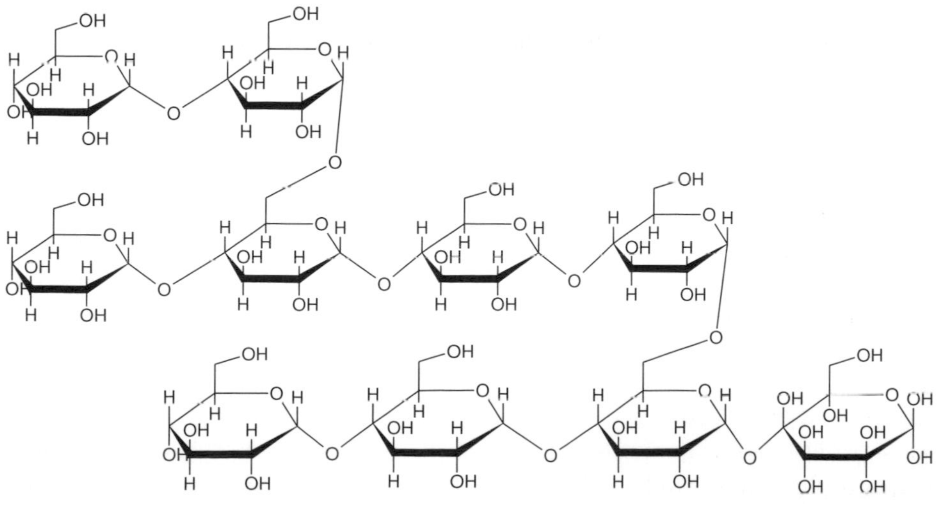

soluble and readily digestible. If cooked starch is then allowed to cool, some of the amylose will adopt a crystalline structure, with neighbouring molecules aligned in the same plane forming hydrogen bonds. This so-called retrograded amylose is then somewhat less readily digested by amylase enzymes.

4.2.4.2 Glycogen

Carbohydrate is stored in animals as glycogen, a molecule with a similar structure to amylopectin. There is very little glycogen in the human diet since it is rapidly lost by glycolysis after death, but oysters eaten live do contain 6 per cent glycogen.

Glycogen is a polymer of glucose and is found in animals

The adult human body can store about 90 g glycogen in the liver plus 350 g in muscle. Thus the total carbohydrate store is equivalent to approximately 1,700 kcal (7 MJ), which is barely one day's energy expenditure. Glycogen is stored with twice its own weight of water, so it would be very heavy to carry much greater carbohydrate stores. Liver glycogen is used to keep blood glucose levels constant (in order to keep the brain functioning) during a short-term fast, for example between meals, and is replenished after the next meal. Muscle glycogen can't release glucose into the bloodstream, so is only used locally to fuel exercise. It becomes depleted after heavy or prolonged exercise, and so has to be repleted afterwards from dietary carbohydrate.

Athletes have learned that if muscles are depleted of glycogen, by exercising to exhaustion, and a low carbohydrate diet is consumed for the next 1–3 days, and after this a high carbohydrate diet is then eaten the muscles will deposit more glycogen than normal. This temporary supercompensation phenomenon is known as glycogen loading, and can enhance the athlete's performance during an event such as a marathon run immediately afterwards.

■ 4.2.5 DIETARY FIBRE (NON-STARCH POLYSACCHARIDES)

These terms are used more or less interchangeably to cover several different classes of substances which share the common feature of being indigestible by the enzymes of the human gut. They are all derived from plants, where they have mainly structural and protective functions. Indeed, the original definition of dietary fibre referred specifically to plant cell walls. The term 'unavailable carbohydrate' is also sometimes used, though the older term 'roughage' is now considered unscientific.

The confusion generated by the different terminology is exacerbated by the existence of several different analytical techniques for their measurement, all of which produce different values. In food tables in the UK values for dietary fibre are obtained using the Southgate method (Southgate, 1969), while those for non-starch polysaccharides are obtained using the Englyst method (Englyst et al., 1982). Values for dietary fibre are generally about 50 per cent higher than values for non-starch polysaccharide content

Unavailable carbohydrate includes celluloses, hemicelluloses, pectic substances and lignin

of the same food. The AOAC method is now being introduced for food tables; this gives slightly higher values than the Englyst method because it includes non-digestible oligosaccharides (AOAC, 2000).

4.2.5.1 Celluloses

These are high molecular weight polymers of glucose joined by $1-4_\beta$ links and arranged in long straight chains, with much hydrogen bonding between adjacent molecules. This makes them physically strong and very insoluble: they need to be dispersed in concentrated sulphuric acid which is then diluted to achieve hydrolysis. Cellulose is characteristically present in all plant cell walls, though it is not necessarily the major component. Celluloses are not digested by amylase, but bacterial cellulases will degrade them. Thus they are extensively fermented in the rumen, though not to any great extent in the human colon.

4.2.5.2 Hemicelluloses
This is a heterogeneous group of non-cellulosic polysaccharides that are insoluble in water but soluble in alkaline solutions of various strengths. It includes polymers of a number of sugars other than glucose, often including uronic acids. They undergo limited fermentation in the colon.

4.2.5.3 Pectic substances
These are characteristically found in fruits, but also in most legumes and in some cereals (e.g. oats). They are soluble in hot water, and are known to food scientists and home economists as thickening and gelling agents. Some are extracted to be used as food additives for these purposes, and may be given specific names including gums, such as guar and tragacanth, and mucilages, such as ispaghula. Alginates are similar substances extracted from algae. All are extensively fermented in the colon.

4.2.5.4 Lignins
Lignins are classically included as fibre, although chemically they are not carbohydrates but polymers of aromatic alcohols. They are the secondary thickening of plant stems, which is deposited as plants get older. Lignin may become covalently bonded to other polysaccharides, making analysis more difficult and impeding bacterial fermentation. They are chemically and nutritionally very inert.

■ 4.2.6 SUGAR ALCOHOLS
These are found in nature, but are also synthesized commercially for use as sweeteners e.g. isomalt, xylitol and sorbitol; they are also referred to as polyols. They are generally poor substrates for bacterial fermentation in the mouth and thus do not cause acid formation and dental caries. Isomalt and xylitol are used in tooth-friendly sweets and chewing gum. Most polyols are not absorbed in the small intestine and thus enter the colon where they are fermented to varying extents to yield short chain fatty acids and gas. There is a limit to the amounts that can be consumed because they increase osmotic pressure and can cause diarrhoea if consumed in excess.

■ 4.3 CARBOHYDRATE INTAKE
The average intake of carbohydrate in the UK is 250 g/d, representing 42 per cent of energy intake. This consists of 100 g sugars, 130 g starch and 20 g fibre. Bread accounts for one quarter of the available carbohydrate, and other cereal products for another quarter, while potatoes account for another 10 per cent. Half the fibre also comes from cereal products, and most of the rest comes from vegetables, particularly legumes, with less than 10 per cent coming from fruit.

Carbohydrate forms an even greater proportion of the diet in poorer countries, since as people become more affluent they tend to replace carbohydrate with fat. Thus carbohydrate accounts for nearly 80 per cent of energy in African diets as a whole, and at least 65 per cent in Caribbean diets, but less than 50 per cent in European and North American diets. Starch is always the major carbohydrate, and much of it is from 'staple foods' (the most abundant item in the average diet of a community). On average 85 per cent of carbohydrate comes from staple foods in developing countries, compared with 62 per cent in developed countries.

Starch is the most abundant carbohydrate in all human diets

■ 4.4 DIGESTION AND ABSORPTION

Starch digestion begins in the mouth with the action of the salivary amylase, ptyalin. It then ceases in the stomach because of the low pH. Most digestion then occurs in the duodenum, where the pH rises again and pancreatic amylase is secreted. This enzyme breaks alternate $1-4_\alpha$ bonds, producing maltose, maltotriose and limit dextrins, which are small oligosaccharide remnants from the branching points in amylopectin molecules.

The products of luminal digestion are hydrolysed further at the brush border of the intestinal mucosa, where glucosidases can hydrolyse the dextrins and maltase hydrolyses the maltose to glucose. Glucose is then absorbed both by diffusion and by an active transport mechanism which requires sodium and ATP. From the mucosal cells glucose can diffuse down a concentration gradient into portal blood.

There are similar disaccharidase enzymes, sucrase and lactase, in the mucosal membrane to hydrolyse sucrose and lactose to their constituent monosaccharides, and these are absorbed by the same mechanisms as glucose.

Absorption of sugars is normally very efficient, except in the case of acquired lactose intolerance. In many people, particularly those of African, Asian or Middle Eastern ethnic origin, lactase activity is lost after the ages of early childhood. This is not surprising, since until recently (in evolutionary terms) it was rare for anyone other than infants and young children to drink milk. The consequences of lactose intolerance are that ingested lactose stays in the lumen of the gut, drawing water in. Some is fermented to lactic acid, drawing more water in which causes diarrhoea, and gases (hydrogen and methane) which are responsible for flatulence, distension and pain. Thus individuals who are lactose intolerant learn to avoid consuming more than a small amount of milk, even though this deprives their diet of a valuable source of calcium and protein.

■ 4.4.1 RESISTANT STARCH

Cooked starch has classically been considered to be rapidly and completely digestible, but recent work has focused attention on differences in the rate and extent of digestion of starch in different foodstuffs. Digestibility can be measured by incubating the food *in vitro* with pancreatic amylase, and this has revealed that most cooked starch is completely hydrolysed within 20 minutes, and is thus classified as readily digestible starch. Even milled raw cereals (flour), together with a proportion of the starch in pasta, are completely digested within two hours, and this fraction has been called slowly digestible starch.

Any starch that is undigested after two hours is called resistant starch. This includes raw cereal grains and other seeds that have been only partly milled, in which significant amounts of starch are still enclosed in indigestible, fibrous seed coats which prevent the access of digestive enzymes. It also includes raw potato and banana starch which is enclosed in indigestible granules. The third category of resistant starch is the retrograded amylose which forms when cooked potato or cereal starch is allowed to cool and recrystallize. It should be noted, however, that the resistant starch content of the starch in most foods is considerably less than 5 per cent, so that starch can still be considered to be at least 95 per cent digestible.

> The digestibility of starch in human diets is around 95 per cent

■ 4.4.2 FERMENTATION OF FIBRE IN THE COLON

The non-starch polysaccharides, together with any resistant starch and undigested oligosaccharides, pass through the small intestine and into the colon. Here there is a massive population of bacteria which are able to ferment many types of carbohydrate. Soluble carbohydrates such as pectin can be completely fermented, whereas insoluble polysaccharides such as cellulose undergo very limited degradation, especially if they are also associated with lignin.

The main products of fermentation are the short chain fatty acids acetate, propionate and butyrate, together with the gases carbon dioxide, hydrogen and methane. The proportions of the different products formed depends on the nature of the substrates entering the colon and the proportions of the different bacteria present. For example, the fermentation of starch produces a high proportion of butyrate while pectin produces very little butyrate.

> Fermentation of undigested carbohydrate in the colon produces acetate, propionate, butyrate, CO_2, H_2 and CH_4

The short chain fatty acids are absorbed from the colon. Propionate is metabolized to release energy, or for gluconeogenesis, in the liver, while acetate is used as a fuel both by the liver and peripheral tissues. Butyrate is the preferred fuel substrate for colonocytes, where it is metabolized to acetoacetate and β-hydroxybutyrate. Thus a considerable proportion of the energy from unavailable carbohydrates may actually be available to the body, and data from studies feeding mixed sources of fibre have suggested that a metabolizable energy value of 8 kJ/g (2 kcal/g) may be appropriate.

• **Figure 4.4** Fermentation of unavailable carbohydrates in the colon

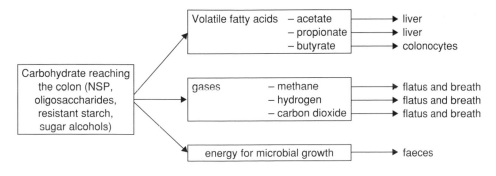

The gases which are produced during colonic fermentation may also be absorbed across the wall of the colon and ultimately expired in the breath. Indeed measurement of increased levels of hydrogen in the breath can be used to indicate the arrival of unavailable carbohydrate in the colon. However when the capacity of the colon to absorb gases is exceeded the excess is passed as flatus.

■ 4.5 METABOLISM OF A GLUCOSE LOAD

Glucose is used in the body for energy, or stored as glycogen or converted to fat

Most carbohydrate enters the bloodstream as glucose for transport to the tissues, where it has three possible metabolic fates: it can be used for energy, stored as glycogen in the liver and muscles, or converted to fat.

■ 4.5.1 FUEL

Glucose can be metabolized as a source of energy via glycolysis and, so long as the supply of oxygen is adequate, the tricarboxylic acid cycle. If there is insufficient oxygen, entry to the tricarboxylic acid cycle is blocked and the end-product of glycolysis, pyruvate, is converted to lactate.

Most tissues will utilize glucose as an energy source after a meal, then switch progressively to fatty acids. The main exception is the liver, which oxidizes very little glucose. Its main fuels are short chain fatty acids and amino acids. In contrast, some tissues have an obligatory need for glucose. In the case of the brain, which is the biggest user of circulating glucose, this is because the fatty acids can't get across the blood-brain barrier. Tissues such as the lens of the eye and the red blood cells are unable to oxidize fatty acids because they have no mitochondria. In other cases, such as the kidney medulla and the skin, fatty acids cannot be oxidized because of poor oxygen delivery.

■ 4.5.2 STORAGE AS GLYCOGEN

Glycogen is stored in muscle, to replace what has been used for exercise, and in the liver, for subsequent use to maintain blood glucose. It should be noted that most glycogen synthesized in the liver after a meal is made from lactate, via a so-called indirect pathway which involves the enzymes of gluconeogenesis. This is because the affinity of glucokinase for glucose is very low, so that the liver does not take up significant amounts of glucose from the circulation unless the glucose concentration exceeds 15 mM. This allows tissues such as the brain to have priority in taking up glucose.

■ 4.5.3 CONVERSION TO FAT

Glucose can be converted to fatty acids and glycerol phosphate in both liver and adipose tissue, and these components are made into triacylglycerols. Triacylglycerols which are synthesized in the liver are secreted as very low density lipoproteins and transported to adipose tissue for storage. Recent evidence suggests that very little fatty acid is synthesized *de novo* in humans, and that most of the fat that is stored comes from dietary fat, but this may simply reflect the relatively high fat content of the mixed diets which most people consume.

■ 4.5.4 CONTROL OF BLOOD GLUCOSE

Clearance of glucose is under the control of the hormone insulin, which is secreted in response to glucose absorption. Insulin facilitates both glucose transport and its utilization in muscle and adipose tissue, and suppresses gluconeogenesis in the liver.

Postabsorbtively, insulin levels fall, preventing glucose uptake into muscle and adipose tissue, thereby ensuring that it is available for uptake by the brain.

■ 4.6 EFFECTS OF UNAVAILABLE CARBOHYDRATE INTAKE ON HEALTH

Many epidemiological studies have shown an inverse relationship between habitual fibre intakes and the incidence of certain diseases, notably coronary heart disease, colon cancer, diverticular disease, appendicitis, gallstones, varicose veins, hiatus hernia, haemorrhoids, obesity and diabetes. In many cases increased fibre intake is also beneficial in their treatment. These are all multifactorial diseases: fibre content is only one aspect of the diet that may be involved in their aetiology, and other environmental and genetic factors are also involved. Some of the mechanisms by which dietary fibre may influence the development of these diseases are set out below.

■ 4.6.1 FOOD INTAKE

Food intake tends to be reduced on bulky, high fibre diets. One possible mechanism is that such diets require more chewing, causing more saliva and more gastric juice to be secreted, which in turn causes greater stomach distension and slower gastric emptying, and thus an earlier or greater feeling of satiety. It may also be that high fibre diets are less tasty than diets with a higher concentration of fat and sugar, and thus less likely to induce overeating, or that too much fibre causes bloating and flatulence, and the discomfort puts people off eating too much.

Fibre tends to delay gastric emptying and slow down glucose absorption

■ 4.6.2 GLUCOSE ABSORPTION

The presence of fibre reduces the rate of gastric emptying, so food enters the small intestine more slowly and thus glucose is absorbed more slowly. Also, once the digesta reaches the small intestine the higher viscosity caused by soluble fibres, especially gums, slows the diffusion of nutrients to the gut wall, so again glucose is absorbed more slowly. The presence of intact remnants of plant cell walls may also inhibit the access of digestive enzymes to starch, thereby slowing its digestion. The decreased rate of glucose absorption is useful for treating Type II diabetes. It has also been suggested that this may help prevent diabetes and heart disease, by reducing insulin secretion. Periodic high peaks of insulin secretion are thought to contribute to the aetiology of both diseases.

The term 'glycaemic index' is now used to describe the rate and extent of the rise in blood glucose following a meal (see Box 4.1). The glycaemic index of a food is defined as the ratio of the area under the blood glucose curve following ingestion of a portion of that food containing 50 g of available carbohydrate to the area under the blood glucose curve following the ingestion of a portion of white bread or glucose containing the same amount of available carbohydrate. As well as its soluble fibre content, the glycaemic index of a food is affected by its content of sugar (since on digestion sucrose produces only half as much glucose as the same amount of starch), the degree of gelatinization of starch, and the presence of any structural components that may hinder the access of digestive enzymes. It is also affected by the other components, including protein and fat, within the food or meal.

BOX 4.1 CALCULATION OF GLYCAEMIC INDEX

Glycaemic index is determined by feeding healthy volunteers a portion of the food being tested containing 50 g of glucose and measuring blood glucose concentration at 15 minute intervals for the next two hours. A blood glucose curve such as the ones below is then drawn, and the area under the curve is calculated. On another occasion the same volunteers are fed a portion of spaghetti containing 50 g of available carbohydrate and the same measurements are made. Glycaemic index is calculated as the ratio of the area under the second blood glucose curve to that of the first. In the example shown the glycaemic index is 41 per cent.

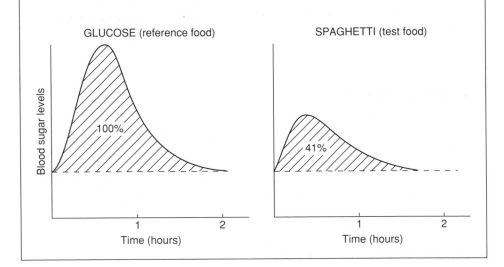

■ 4.6.3 FAECAL BULK

The presence of undigested carbohydrate residues draws water into the lumen of the large intestine, considerably increasing faecal mass. This also increases the rate at which the faeces pass through the colon, i.e. it decreases the transit time. This helps to relieve constipation, which is important in itself for many people, and it also helps to prevent other diseases which may be caused by the high intra-abdominal pressure which results from straining to void small hard faeces. These diseases include hiatus hernia, haemorrhoids and varicose veins, which may result from inhibition of the venous return from the legs by high intra-abdominal pressure. The greater faecal mass also helps to dilute potential carcinogens and other toxins, and the more rapid transit through the colon reduces the length of time for which they are in contact with the intestinal wall, thereby reducing the risk of colon cancer. Some of the sources of dietary fibre (e.g. pectin and β-glucans) are able to bind to bile acids, preventing their reabsorption and promoting their excretion in faeces. To compensate for the increased loss of bile acids in faeces, further bile acids are synthesized from cholesterol in the liver, and the reduction in the hepatic cholesterol pool causes an upregulation of LDL receptors which results in a reduction in plasma cholesterol concentration (see Chapter 9 for further discussion on the regulation of plasma cholesterol concentrations).

Fibre increases faecal bulk and decreases transit time

■ 4.6.4 BACTERIAL FERMENTATION

As described earlier there is a large mass of bacteria within the colon which utilizes undigested carbohydrate as its main energy source. These bacteria can detoxify some carcinogens. The butyric acid produced by bacterial fermentation tends to stimulate cell division in the gut mucosa, but apparently without stimulating neoplastic growth. Another product of bacterial fermentation is propionic acid, some of which is absorbed and can inhibit cholesterol synthesis in the liver. However, acetic acid which is also produced from some substrates stimulates cholesterol synthesis.

Finally it should be noted that some of these effects are not confined to dietary fibre but also apply to resistant starch and oligosaccharides. Consequently, dietary advice now focuses on promoting the health benefits of foods rich in complex carbohydrates rather than specifically advocating dietary fibre.

SUMMARY

- Dietary carbohydrates fall into three main groups: sugars, starch and non-starch polysaccharides (dietary fibre).
- The main sugar in the diet is sucrose which accounts for around 14 per cent of energy intake. Sucrose intake should be limited because of its deleterious effect on dental health.
- Starch is a polymer of glucose which accounts for over a quarter of our energy intake.
- Dietary fibre refers to a series of substances that are not digested in the human small intestine, including cellulose and hemicellulose, gums and pectins.
- Available carbohydrates enter the body as glucose which can be oxidized to produce energy, stored as glycogen or converted to fat.
- Unavailable carbohydrates remain in the intestine, and some can be fermented by colonic bacteria to produce volatile fatty acids and gases.
- A high intake of complex carbohydrates and dietary fibre has a number of health benefits.

FURTHER READING

British Nutrition Foundation (1990) *Complex Carbohydrates in Foods. The Report of the British Nutrition Foundation's Task Force*. London: Chapman and Hall.

Department of Health and Social Security (1989) *Dietary Sugars and Human Disease. Report of the Panel on Dietary Sugars*. London: HMSO.

Englyst, H., Wiggins, H.S. and Cummings, J.H. (1982) 'Determination of non-starch polysaccharides in plant foods by gas-liquid chromatography of constituent sugars as alditol acetates', *Analyst*, 107: 307–18.

FAO/WHO (Joint) (1998) *Expert consultation on carbohydrates in human nutrition*. Rome: FAO/WHO.

Association of Official Analytical Chemists (2000) *Official Methods of Analysis*, 17th edn.

Southgate, D.A.T. (1969) 'Determination of carbohydrates in foods: II Unavailable carbohydrates', *J. Sci. Fd. Agric.*, 20: 331–5.

■ 5.1 INTRODUCTION

Fat has come to be regarded as an undesirable constituent of human diets. It has been linked to obesity and cardiovascular disease (discussed in Chapter 9) but it does play an important role in meeting nutrient requirements, and certain types of fat offer protection from heart disease. This chapter discusses the need for fat in the diet, in particular its role in supplying energy, enabling the absorption of fat-soluble nutrients, and the provision of essential fatty acids.

■ 5.2 THE CHEMISTRY OF FATS

The term fat is used to describe fatty acids and fatty acid esters. Fat in food used to be measured by the Soxhlet method which determined the amount of material that was soluble in organic solvents such as petroleum ether. However, this crude method also measured other non-polar material. Nowadays, the fat content of food is determined by gas liquid chromatography (GLC). In this process, free and esterified fatty acids are first converted to volatile derivatives, usually methyl esters, and then separated by GLC according to chain length and unsaturation.

The term lipid is now preferred to fat. According to Christie (2002), 'Lipids are fatty acids and their derivatives, and substances related biosynthetically or functionally to these compounds.' He goes on to define fatty acids as 'compounds synthesised in nature via condensation of malonyl coenzyme A units by a fatty acid synthase complex. They usually contain even numbers of carbon atoms in straight chains (commonly C14 to C24), and may be saturated or unsaturated, and can contain a variety of substituent groups.'

The most common lipid classes in nature consist of fatty acids linked by an ester bond to glycerol (triacylglycerols, diacylglycerols, monoacylglycerols or phosphoglycerides), or to other alcohols such as cholesterol (cholesteryl esters) or sphingoid bases (sphingolipids). Dietary fat consists mainly of triacylglycerols. Fatty acids can be at one of three positions: $sn-1$, $sn-2$ and $sn-3$. Phosphoglycerides are related compounds but have a phosphate

• **Figure 5.1** Major body lipids

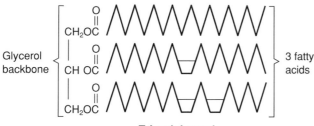

Triacylglycerol
Main constituent of dietary fats used
for energy storage in adipose tissue

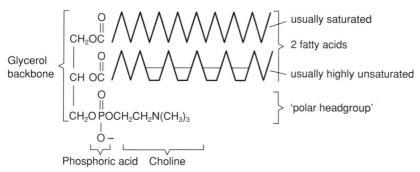

Glycerol backbone

usually saturated

2 fatty acids

usually highly unsaturated

'polar headgroup'

Phosphoric acid   Choline

Phospholipid
Used as structural component in membranes
and can donate fatty acid to form eicosanoids

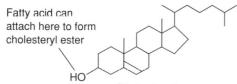

Fatty acid can
attach here to form
cholesteryl ester

Cholesterol
Membrane component and also precursor of bile acids,
vitamin D and steroid hormones

group and a polar head group (choline, ethanolamine, inositol or serine) at the *sn* − 3 position (Figure 5.1).

Fatty acids consist of a carbon backbone terminated by a carboxyl group (COOH) at one end and a methyl group (CH_3) at the other. Fatty acids differ with regard to their chain length, unsaturation and position and geometry (*cis* or *trans*) of their double bonds (Figure 5.2). Fatty acid chain length can vary from 2 to more than 80 carbon atoms but most commonly they are 14, 16, 18, 20 and 22 carbon atoms long. Odd and branched chain fatty acids are less common and are generally of microbial origin. They are present in small amounts in dairy, beef and lamb fat and in fats from the marine food chain (from algae). These branched chain fatty acids are generally not of any nutritional significance except among individuals with an inborn error of metabolism called Refsum's Disease

cis configuration

trans configuration

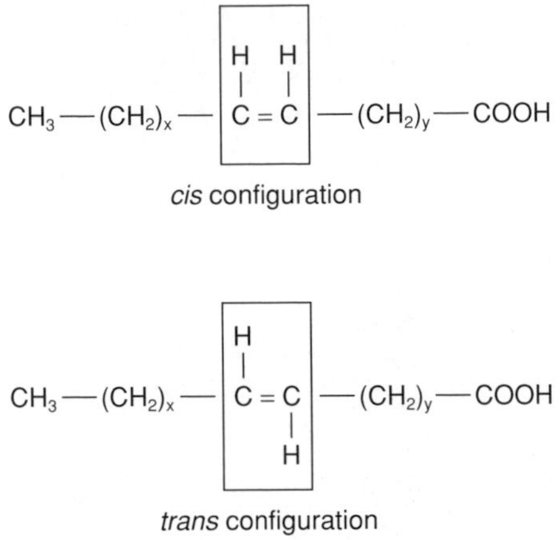

who are unable to oxidize branched fatty acids. Table 5.1 gives a list of the fatty acids commonly found in nature, their sources and the shorthand structure used to describe them. Fatty acids can be divided into saturated and unsaturated fatty acids (Figure 5.2).

■ 5.2.1 SATURATED FATTY ACIDS

Fatty acids in which all the carbon atoms in the chain are linked by single bonds are called saturated fatty acids. Most dietary saturated fatty acids are 12–18 carbon atoms long and solid at room temperature (25 °C) and relatively insoluble in water. Palmitic acid (16:0) is the most commonly occurring dietary saturated fatty acid. Short chain saturated fatty acids (sometimes referred to as volatile fatty acids) are 2–6 carbon atoms long (acetic, butyric and valeric), and are relatively water soluble. They are produced by bacterial fermentation of carbohydrates and are present in cow's milk and butter. Medium chain saturated fatty acids 8–12 carbon atoms long are found in some tropical oils such as coconut oil and palm kernel oil and are liquid at room temperature and partially soluble in water.

■ 5.2.2 UNSATURATED FATTY ACIDS

Unsaturated fatty acids contain one or more double bonds at specific positions in the carbon chain and are most commonly 16–22 carbon atoms long. Double bonds can exist in two forms or configurations: *cis* and *trans*; the most common is the *cis* form (Figure 5.2) where both hydrogen atoms are on the same side of the double bond. The insertion of a *cis* double bond puts a kink in the molecule and this lowers the melting point of the fatty acid.

Unsaturated fatty acids can be further subdivided into two groups: those with one double bond are called **monounsaturated** and those with two or more double bonds are called **polyunsaturated** (Figure 5.3). Specific enzymes called **desaturases**, present in plants and animals, can insert a *cis* double bond in a saturated fatty acid by removing two hydrogen atoms from an adjacent pair of carbons.

Plant desaturase enzymes insert double bonds at positions 3, 6 and 9 from the terminal methyl group whereas animal desaturases are only capable of inserting double bonds at specific positions in the carbon chain beyond position 6 from the terminal methyl group.

Table 5.1 Major fatty acids on plant and animal origin

Systematic name	Trivial name	Shorthand†	Significant dietary sources
Saturated			
ethanoic	acetic	2:0	butter
butanoic	butyric	4:0	butter
hexanoic	caproic	6:0	butter
octanoic	caprylic	8:0	goat's milk
decanoic	capric	10:0	goat's milk
dodecanoic	lauric	12:0	coconut oil
tetradecanoic	myristic	14:0	coconut oil, animal fats
hexadecanoic	palmitic	16:0	palm oil, animal fats
octadecanoic	stearic	18:0	cocoabutter, hydrogenated fats
eicosanoic	arachidic	20:0	peanuts
docosanoic	behenic	22:0	
Monounsaturated			
cis-9-hexadecenoic	palmitoleic	$16:1n-7$	fish oil
cis-6-octadecenoic	petroselinic	$18:1n-12$	
cis-9-octadecenoic	oleic	$18:1n-9$	olive oil, rapeseed oil, palm oil
trans-9-octadecenoic	elaidic	$18:1n-9trans$	partially hydrogenated fats
trans-11-octadecenoic	trans-vaccenic	$18:1n-7trans$	ruminant fats
cis-11-octadecenoic	cis-vaccenic	$18:1n-7$	ruminant fats
cis-13-docosenoic	erucic	$22:1n-9$	rapeseed and mustard seed oils
cis-15-tetracosenoic	nervonic	$24:1n-9$	
Polyunsaturated*			
9,12-octadecadienoic	linoleic	$18:2n-6$	safflower, sunflower, corn oil
6,9,12-octadecatrienoic	gamma-linolenic	$18:3n-6$	evening primrose oil
9,12,15-octadecatrienoic	alpha-linolenic	$18:3n-3$	flaxseed oil
8,11,14-eicosatrienoic	dihomogammalinolenic	$20:3n-6$	
5,8,11,14-eicosatetraenoic	arachidonic	$20:4n-6$	
5,8,11,14,17-eicosapentaenoic	eicosapentaenoic	$20:5n-3$	fish oil
4,7,10,13,16,19-docosahexaenoic	docosahexaenoic	$22:6n-3$	fish oil

Notes:
*denotes all cis methylene interrupted
†The number before the colon indicates the number of carbon atoms in the fatty acids, the number after the colon indicates the number of double bonds, n-m indicates the position of the first double bond from the terminal methyl group.

The most abundant monounsaturated fatty acid is oleic acid ($18:1n-9$). It is the major fatty acid in olive oil and rapeseed oil but it is present in large amounts in most oils and fats. Other monounsaturated fatty acids found in food, especially oily fish, are 16, 20 and 22 carbon atoms long. Erucic acid ($22:1n-9$) used to be a major constituent of rapeseed oil and when fed to young animals causes damage to heart muscle. Modern

• **Figure 5.3** Non-essential and essential fatty acid structures

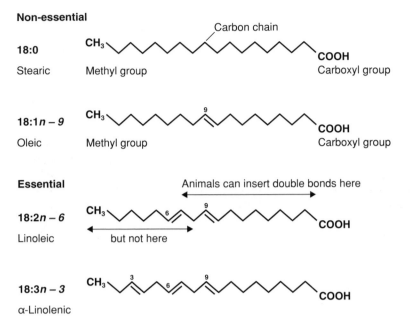

varieties of rapeseed oil (canola) contain negligible amounts of erucic acid and can safely be consumed. The older varieties of rapeseed oil, which are rich in erucic acid, are banned from human consumption in many countries. Mustard seed oil, which is similarly rich in erucic acid, is still used in parts of India and Bangladesh.

■ 5.2.3 *TRANS* FATTY ACIDS

Most unsaturated fatty acids in nature have their double bonds in the *cis* configuration. However, certain bacteria can convert *cis* unsaturated fatty acids into fatty acids with their double bonds in the *trans* configuration where the hydrogen atoms are on the opposite side of the carbon chain. This occurs in ruminants (e.g. cows, sheep and goats) where bacterial fermentation occurs in the rumen (forestomach) leading to the formation of *trans* unsaturated fatty acids. About 4–7 per cent of the fats from the meat and milk of ruminant animals are *trans* fatty acids. *Trans* unsaturated fatty acids are also produced during the industrial hardening of fats using a process called partial hydrogenation. Among the major products of partial hydrogenation of vegetable oils are stearic acid (18:0) and *trans* isomers of 18:1 such as elaidic acid (18:1$n-9$, *trans*). A *trans* double bond does not cause the carbon chain to kink to the same extent as *cis* double bonds and in many respects a monounsaturated fatty acid with a *trans* double bond has characteristics similar to a saturated fatty acid of the same chain length. A *trans* monounsaturated fatty acid has a high melting point nearer that of the saturated fatty acid of the same chain length. For example the melting points of stearic acid (18:0), elaidic acid (18:1$n-9$, *trans*) and oleic acid (18:1$n-9$, *cis*) are 69.6, 44 and 13.2 °C respectively. Partially hydrogenated fats typically contain 5–30 per cent *trans* fatty acids. A high intake of *trans* fatty acids has been associated with increased risk of cardiovascular disease. Consequently, many food manufacturers are seeking ways of decreasing levels in food by avoiding the use of partial hydrogenation.

• **Figure 5.4** Metabolism of essential fatty acids

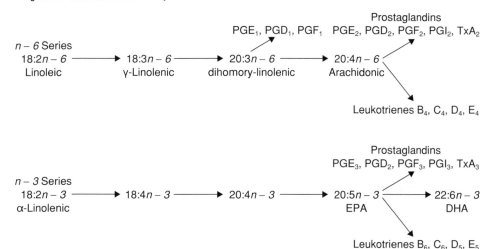

5.2.4 ESSENTIAL FATTY ACIDS

The essential fatty acids are a class of polyunsaturated fatty acids which cannot be made in the body but are required in the diet to promote normal physiological functioning. There are two families of essential fatty acids, the $n-6$ and $n-3$, derived from linoleic acid ($18:2n-6$) and α-linolenic acid ($18:3n-3$) respectively, and they are not interconvertible (Figure 5.4). The position of the first double bond is denoted by $n-3$, if it is 3 carbon atoms from the terminal methyl group, $n-6$ if it is 6 carbon atoms from the carboxyl group. The conversion to longer chain derivatives involves alternating desaturation followed by chain elongation and the double bonds are methylene interrupted. Two desaturase with specificity for inserting double bond at positions Δ6 and Δ5 from the carboxyl end of the fatty acids have been identified and are called Δ6 and Δ5 desaturase respectively.

Mammals are unable to insert double bonds in fatty acids beyond the sixth carbon atom from the terminal methyl group

5.2.4.1 *n* – *6* fatty acids

Linoleic acid ($18:2n-6$) is synthesized in plants and is the dominant fatty acid in many seeds. It is the major fatty acid in sunflower, safflower, corn and soybean oils. Linoleic acid itself plays a very specific role in maintaining the water-permeability barrier in the skin and is also necessary for the normal differentiation of skin cells. It undergoes metabolism to form hydroxy derivatives that appear to regulate gene expression by acting on the PPAR (Peroxysome Proliferator Activated Receptor) nuclear hormone receptor and some of these are constituents of acylglycosylceramides that make up the permeability barrier of the skin. It is converted via γ-linolenic acid and dihomo-gammalinolenic acid to arachidonic acid ($20:4n-6$) in mammalian tissues. Arachidonic acid is an important constituent of most phospholipids that make up cell membranes and is involved in cell signalling (the phosphatidyl inositol signalling pathway and eicosanoid synthesis – see below). Dietary arachidonic acid is found preformed in small amounts in egg yolk and meat. Δ6 desaturase is the rate limiting enzyme in the synthesis of arachidonic acid.

Linoleic acid has a specific role in cholesterol transport and maintaining the normal water barrier of the skin and differentiation of skin cells.

5.2.4.2 n – 3 fatty acids

α-Linolenic acid (18:3$n-3$) is the parent fatty acid of the $n-3$ series. In plants it is syn-thesized by chloroplasts, and monogastric herbivores such as horses and rabbits have high intakes from eating grass. It is found in variable concentrations in vegetable oils but flaxseed, rapeseed and soybean oils contain substantial amounts.

α-Linolenic acid can be converted to eicosapentaenoic acid (20:5$n-3$; EPA) and then docosahexaenoic acid (22:6$n-3$; DHA) in the body. DHA is the major metabolite found in human tissues where it is concentrated in the membrane phospholipids, especially of the retina and brain. Until recently it was believed that DHA was synthesized by the action of a Δ4 desaturase on 22:5$n-3$ but is now believed to occur by an indirect route which involves chain elongation of 20:5$n-3$ to 24:5$n-3$ followed by Δ6 desaturation to form 24:6$n-3$ followed by peroxysomal chain shortening to 22:6$n-3$. The capacity to synthesize DHA from α-linolenic acid appears limited and preformed DHA appears to be required in the diet of the preterm infant. EPA and DHA are also synthesized by a different metabolic route in marine algae that involves the polyketide synthase pathway. EPA and DHA derived from algae accumulate in the marine food chain and this is why relatively high concentrations are found in fish oil.

■ 5.3 COMPOSITION OF DIFFERENT DIETARY FATS

Dietary fats and oils consist mainly of triacylglycerols (TAGs) with smaller amounts of phospholipids and sterol esters. The nature of a TAG is determined by its fatty acid constituents and the position of the fatty acids on the TAG molecule: it can consist of one type of fatty acid or mixtures of different fatty acids. As a rule, TAGs rich in *cis* monounsaturated or polyunsaturated fatty acids tend to be liquid at room temperature (up to 25 °C), for example olive oil, sunflower oil, rapeseed oil and fish oil, whereas those rich in saturated or *trans* fatty acids tend to be solid at room temperature (e.g. butter, tallow, palm oil and partially hydrogenated fats).

Generally plant oils have a symmetrical TAG structure; for example in cocoabutter and palm oil, saturated fatty acids are in positions *sn-1* and *sn-3* and an unsaturated fatty acid such as oleic acid is in the *sn-2* position. This configuration results in a fat with a lower melting point than the asymmetric TAG with saturated fatty acids in the *sn-1* and *sn-2* positions and the unsaturated fatty acids in the *sn-3* position. A good example is cocoabutter where the dominant TAG species is 1,3 distearyl-2-oleyl glycerol. This TAG structure gives chocolate its characteristic texture and feel in the mouth and results in a rapid melting curve at body temperature. Randomizing the structure of cocoabutter increases the melting point and decreases the absorption. The technique of randomization is now being widely used in the food industry as an alternative to partial hydrogenation to produce fats of a higher melting point.

■ 5.4 THE DIGESTION OF FAT

Fat poses a number of problems for its digestion and absorption as it is not soluble in water. In the newborn, fat digestion begins in the stomach, as the infant has the capacity to secrete lipases (enzymes that digest fat) in its saliva and in the stomach. In adults, however, food first has to be emulsified before digestion can occur (Figure 5.5). This is facilitated by the secretion of bile from the gallbladder. Bile acts as a detergent making

• **Figure 5.5** Digestion and absorption of dietary fat

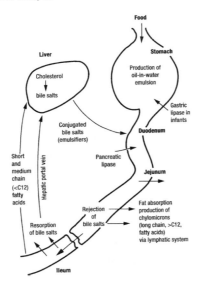

the fat form into small micelles which are soluble in water. These can then be acted on by lipases which are secreted from the pancreas into the gut.

Pancreatic lipase cleaves fatty acids from the *sn-1* and *sn-3* positions of the TAG. The end-products of the digestion of fat are glycerol, fatty acids and 2-monoacylglycerol (MAG), which are absorbed by diffusion across the gut wall. Short-medium-chain fatty acids are relatively water-soluble and after diffusing across the gut wall can be transported to the liver via the hepatic portal vein, bound to albumin. Long chain fatty acids (>12 carbons long) are re-esterified into triacylglycerols which in turn are packaged into lipoprotein particles called chylomicrons. These are transported by the lymphatic system and secreted into the peripheral circulation. About 2–3 hours following a fatty meal, the blood plasma appears cloudy due to the appearance of the chylomicrons. Chylomicrons acquire apolipoprotein C from HDL which is a cofactor for the activation of the enzyme lipoprotein lipase, which is expressed on endothelial cells. The lipoprotein lipase cleaves the fatty acids which are then transported into tissues for storage or metabolism. The lipid-depleted chylomicron remnant is then removed by specific receptors in the liver. Fat-soluble vitamins (vitamins A, E, D and K) and cholesterol are delivered directly to the liver as part of the chylomicron remnants (Figure 5.6).

Digestibility of fat is normally greater than 95 per cent. However, some high melting point TAGs such as tristearin are poorly digested. Diseases that impair the secretion of bile, such as biliary obstruction or hepatitis, lead to severe fat malabsorption, as do diseases that influence the secretion of lipase enzymes from the pancreas, such as cystic fibrosis. It follows, therefore, that normal fat digestion is necessary for the absorption of fat-soluble vitamins. Olestra is a synthetic fat which consists of fatty acids esterified onto a sucrose molecule. Olestra is not digested and is sold as a fat substitute in the USA and is used in snack foods such as crisps and corn chips. Olestra inhibits the absorption of β-carotene but does not have effects on other fat-soluble vitamins.

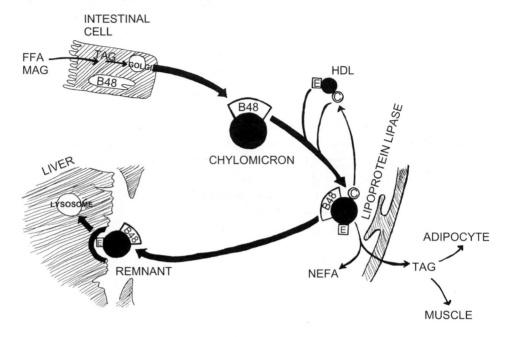

■ 5.5 PHYSIOLOGICAL ROLE OF FAT

■ 5.5.1 FAT AS A SOURCE OF ENERGY

Fatty acids are a major fuel for the body and energy is released by β-oxidation which occurs mainly in the mitochondria. In order that fatty acids can enter the mitochondria, they need to form carnitine esters. However, C20–22 fatty acids do not readily form carnitine esters and undergo β-oxidation outside the mitochondria in peroxysomes. Peroxysomes can be induced by dietary feeding with long chain fatty acids. Short and medium chain fatty acids are more rapidly oxidized to form energy and generate more heat and slightly less ATP than longer chain fatty acids. It has been argued that the presence of medium chain fatty acids in human milk plays an important role in maintaining thermoregulation in the infant.

If energy intake exceeds requirements, the excess is stored as body fat. Fat deposited in adipose tissue usually reflects the composition of dietary fat because other sources of food energy (carbohydrate and alcohol) are preferentially oxidized to supply energy before fat. In humans, there is very little *de novo* synthesis of fatty acids from carbohydrate and alcohol. Alcohol intake increases TAG synthesis mainly by suppressing fatty acid oxidation.

When energy expenditure exceeds energy intake then fat is mobilized from fat stores to provide energy. TAG in adipose tissue is hydrolysed to release non-esterified fatty acids (NEFAs) into the blood where they are transported bound to albumin. NEFAs can be taken up by muscle or liver. NEFAs are the main fuel used by heart muscle and by skeletal muscle during moderate activity. If the rate of conversion of NEFA to acetyl-CoA is greater than the capacity of the tricarboxylic cycle to oxidize acetyl-CoA in the liver, then the excess acetyl-CoA is converted into ketone bodies (acetoacetic acid, β-hydroxybutyrate and acetone). Unlike fatty acids, ketone bodies can be used as a fuel by the brain, thus sparing glucose. The excessive production of ketone bodies can be hazardous because it can cause a metabolic acidosis. However, adaptation does occur after a few days in subjects fed diets that are very high in fat or in subjects on a very low energy intake. If the flux of NEFA into the liver is high and lipid oxidation is suppressed, NEFAs are used to resynthesize TAGs, which are subsequently exported from the liver on very low density lipoproteins (VLDL) (see Chapter 9).

The release of NEFA, and oxidation and synthesis of TAG are under hormonal control and are particularly influenced by adrenaline and insulin. Adrenaline stimulates the release of NEFA from adipose tissue whereas insulin inhibits the release of NEFA and stimulates lipoprotein lipase activity and TAG synthesis.

The fat used by the body is usually a mixture of the fat supplied in the diet and the fat stores. One kilogram of body fat provides approximately 29 MJ, an amount sufficient to support the energy requirements of an adult for about three days. The energy yield of different fats does show some variation. This in turn depends upon the digestibility and fatty acid chain length of the different fats. Elia and Livesey (1992) have estimated the heat of combustion of different fatty acids and established the following predictive equation:

$$\text{Heat of combustion (kJ/mol)} = -1(653n - 166d - 421)$$

where n is the number of carbon atoms/mol fatty acid and d is the number of double bonds per fatty acid.

Short and medium chain fatty acids yield approximately 29 kJ/g and long chain fatty acids yield 37 kJ/g. However, as dietary fats mainly consist of long chain fatty acids, the figure of 37 kJ/g is generally used. Specially manufactured TAG (SALATRIM™) consisting of asymmetric stearic-rich TAG containing propionic and acetic acid has been used to produce fat that supplies 21 kJ/g: the lower enegy value is partly attributed to the high content of short chain fatty acids but is also due to the lower digestibility of the asymmetric stearate-rich TAG.

Adipose tissue also protects and cushions delicate organs, for example the heart and kidneys. The different stores have different rates of turnover with visceral fat, which is located adjacent to the mesenteric vessels in the abdominal cavity, having the highest rate. Subcutaneous fat helps reduce the loss of body heat and this is particularly important in the newborn. Infants have a large surface area relative to their weight and thus a greater surface to lose heat from. Newborn infants are also endowed with brown adipose tissue which has a high capacity to oxidize fat to release energy as heat and this helps them keep warm. It is called brown fat because it contains many mitochondria and has a rich blood supply which gives it a brown colour. It is located around the major arteries on the neck and between the shoulder blades. The mitochondria in brown adipose tissue express uncoupling protein (also called thermogenin) which functions as a proton carrier. It blocks the proton electrochemical gradient and stimulates respiration. The free energy change associated with respiration is dissipated as heat rather than ATP.

Women have more adipose tissue than men but the pattern of fat distribution differs between genders. Fat is deposited mostly under the skin in women, particularly around the hips, whereas in men fat is deposited mainly in the abdomen, between the shoulder blades and around the waist. Typically 18–25 per cent of the weight of a healthy woman is fat, whereas in men only 12–15 per cent is fat. The fat patterning in women is determined by the action of oestrogen and after the menopause, there is redistribution of fat from the hips and thighs to the abdomen.

Body fat in women is an important energy reserve to subsidize the increased energy requirement of pregnancy and lactation. A certain threshold level of body fat of around 18 per cent body weight is necessary to support fertility and the expression of secondary sexual characteristics (development of the breasts and suppression of hair growth on the limbs and face). If the level of body fat drops below about 15 per cent then menstruation ceases. The exact mechanism by which body fat regulates fertility in women is not clearly understood, but it is probably a response to the production of leptin by adipose tissue which has actions on the hypothalamus to stimulate the menstrual cycle.

■ 5.5.2 STRUCTURAL LIPIDS

Structural lipids account for 5–8 per cent of body weight and these are composed mainly of phospholipids and cholesterol, which make up membrane lipids. The essential fatty acids are required as constituents of phospholipids and linoleic acid play an important role in the transport of cholesterol as cholesteryl esters in plasma. Phospholipids generally have polyunsaturated fatty acids in the sn-2 position. There is specificity for certain polyunsaturated fatty acids in some tissues. For example, in platelet membrane lipids arachidonic acid accounts for almost all of the fatty acids in the sn-2 position of phosphatidyl inositol (PI) whereas in ethanolamine phosphoglycerides of the retina, docosahexaenoic acid is the major fatty acid in the sn-2 position. These differences appear to be related to a difference in function. The role of arachidonic acid in PI is to be involved in cell signalling whereas the role of DHA in the retina appears to be associated with facilitating conformational changes in rhodopsin which is embedded in the membrane.

■ 5.5.3 EICOSANOID FORMATION

Oxygenated derivatives of the essential fatty acids are important regulatory signals. The term eicosanoid was coined to describe the various metabolites generated by the enzymic oxidation of C20 polyunsaturated fatty acids. Eicosanoids are formed when the polyunsaturated fatty acid substrate (usually arachidonic acid) is released from a phospholipid usually by the action of phospholipase A2 but also by the combined action of phospholipase C and diacylglycerol lipase. The first class of compounds to be discovered was the prostaglandins which are formed by the action of cyclo-oxygenase. Cyclo-oxygenase exists in two forms: a constitutive form (COX-1), which performs housekeeping duties in cells, and an inducible form (COX-2), which is responsible for causing inflammation. Arachidonic acid is the major substrate for cyclo-oxygenase but other fatty acids such as dihomo-gammalinolenic acid ($20:3n-6$) and EPA are also substrates. EPA and DHA also act as competitive inhibitors of cyclo-oxygenase besides decreasing substrate concentrations of arachidonic acid in the sn-2 position of phospholipids.

The action of cyclo-oxygenase on arachidonic acid results in the formation of a cyclic endoperoxide (PGH_2) which is transformed into prostaglandin derivatives by specific synthases. The pattern of metabolites varies from tissue to tissue depending on which

• **Figure 5.7** Eicosanoid synthesis from arachidonic acid

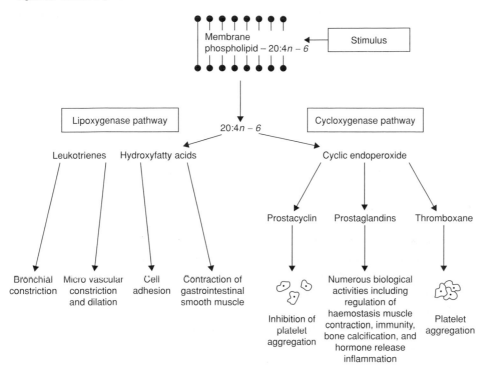

synthases are expressed. Many of the effects of prostaglandins are mediated in concert with the phosphatidyl inositol signalling system and are accompanied by changes in intracellular cyclic AMP concentration. A variety of lipoxygenases are expressed in cells, the 5-lipoxygenase enzyme gives rise to a set of compounds called leukotrienes which are involved in chemotaxis and inflammation. Leukotrienes are produced by leucocytes and by lung cells and they were formerly known as the slow releasing substance of anaphylaxis. As the name implies, they are produced in allergic reactions and they contribute to bronchoconstriction in asthma attacks.

The pattern of eicosanoid metabolites varies between tissues (Figure 5.7). For example, two eicosanoids, thromboxane TxA_2 and prostacyclin PGI_2 are both derived from arachidonic acid but are produced in different locations, the platelets and endothelial cells, and play an important role in haemostasis. When a blood vessel is damaged, platelets stick to the damaged vessel wall and a sequence of reactions occurs, resulting in the release of arachidonic acid from intracellular phospholipids and its conversion to thromboxane TxA_2. This triggers a reduction in intracellular cyclic AMP concentration, resulting in platelet aggregation and degranulation of platelet vesicles, and causes constriction of local blood vessels. Platelet aggregates in turn stimulate blood clot formation, thus stemming the loss of blood in the event of injury. The blood vessel wall responds by synthesizing prostacyclin PGI_2 which inhibits further platelet aggregation by increasing platelet cyclic AMP concentrations and causes vasodilatation; thus localizing blood clot formation to the site of injury. Prostaglandins PGE_2 and $PGF_{2\alpha}$, derived from arachidonic acid, are also involved in initiating uterine contractions during birth. Pregnant rats fed a diet deficient in linoleic acid are unable to give birth to any young conceived, because of failure to produce these prostaglandins. Synthetic prostaglandins are used to induce labour in women.

Prostaglandin PGE_2 is also involved in cell signalling, particularly in cells of the immune system. Many anti-inflammatory drugs act by inhibiting cyclo-oxygenase, e.g. aspirin and paracetamol. One of the known side-effects of aspirin is to trigger attacks of asthma in sensitive individuals. This is believed to occur because arachidonic acid is diverted down the 5-lipoxygenase pathway to form leukotrienes.

Eicosanoid metabolites can be formed from EPA but they are generally inactive (with the exception of prostacyclin PGI_3) or less active than those derived from arachidonic acid. The consumption of EPA results in the displacement of arachidonic acid from membrane lipids and so also reduces the capacity to produce active eicosanoids. This can be used experimentally to decrease inflammatory disorders.

Arachidonic acid which is synthesized from linoleic acid is the major eicosanoid precursor

■ 5.5.4 ROLE OF ESSENTIAL FATTY ACIDS IN GENE TRANSCRIPTION

Certain derivatives of the essential fatty acids are ligands for nuclear hormone receptors. They are ligands for the PPAR and LXR (liver X) receptors which form heterodimers with the RXR (retinoid X) receptor which in turn bind to specific binding element motifs that regulate gene transcription. Prostaglandin J2 and hydroxy metabolites of linoleic acid are ligands for the $PPAR_\gamma$ receptor, which has been shown to regulate the sensitivity of cells to the action of insulin. DHA and EPA are ligands for $PPAR_\alpha$ which induces a switch from lipid synthesis to lipid oxidation in the liver and induces extramitochondrial lipid oxidation in peroxysomes. DHA is also a ligand for the LXR receptor which is involved in the regulation of the efflux of cholesterol from cells via the ATP cassette binding protein type 1 (ABC-1). It has been observed that high intakes of EPA decrease the production of the cytokines TNF_α, $IL-1_\beta$ and IL-6. This could be a consequence of decreased production of prostaglandin PGE_2 and leukotriene LTB_4. However, there is some evidence that EPA may interfere with the activation of NFKappaB, which is a transcription factor involved in regulating the production of inflammatory mediators.

C20–22 polyunsaturated fatty acids are ligands for the $PPAR_\alpha$ and LXR nuclear hormone receptors

■ 5.5.5 MEETING ENERGY REQUIREMENTS

Fat plays an important role in meeting energy requirements. Although the role of fat in providing energy is a hypothetically dispensable one (in that energy can be provided by other nutrients), it is particularly important in providing sufficient energy density in the diets of the very young. Most of the energy in human milk is provided by fat. On average fat supplies 37 kJ/g compared with 16 kJ/g for carbohydrate. Fat provides a concentrated supply of energy and thus reduces the bulk of the diet. The addition of a little fat to food can double its food energy value. Decreasing fat intake can drastically lower energy intake. For example, a 200 ml glass of skimmed milk contains 276 kJ/glass compared with 550 kJ in a 200 ml glass of full cream milk. While a reduction in energy density may be desirable for an individual trying to restrict their energy intake, it can be undesirable for a child under the age of 5-years-old when energy requirements are relatively high, and milk is an important source of energy. There is little doubt that a restricted energy intake is the major factor responsible for poor growth in many developing countries and in this context an increased fat intake is desirable.

On the other hand, diets high in fat are conducive to obesity in adults in part because of their high energy density. It has also been argued that individuals are less able to regulate energy intakes effectively when the diet is high in fat. However, the evidence suggests that a decline in physical activity rather than an increased energy intake is responsible for the increasing prevalence of obesity. Obesity is a complex disorder and restriction of energy intake, especially that supplied by fat, is central to its management (see Chapter 9).

■ 5.5.6 FAT AS A SOLVENT

Fat is an excellent solvent for many organic compounds. It acts as a solvent for flavours and fat-soluble vitamins as well as fat-soluble contaminants. Dietary fats are sources of the fat-soluble vitamins A, D, E and K and are also necessary for the absorption of these compounds. β-carotene, a fat-soluble substance that can be converted into vitamin A in the body, is found in large amounts in carrots, dark green leafy vegetables and yellow/orange fruits (e.g. apricot, mango and papaya), and is poorly absorbed on a low fat diet. In parts of the world such as South East Asia where the intake of fat is very low, vitamin A deficiency disease is common in toddlers. It is estimated that at least 15 per cent of dietary energy needs to be provided as fat to facilitate the absorption of the fat-soluble vitamins. Vitamin A deficiency is almost never seen in developed countries where there is an abundance of good sources of vitamin A such as butter, margarine to which it is added, cheese, full cream milk and eggs. Skimmed milk, low-fat yoghurt and cottage cheese contain virtually no vitamin A. In view of the role of fat in supplying fat-soluble vitamins and energy, it seems that relatively high fat intakes are desirable in the first five years of life.

■ 5.5.7 FAT AND PALATABILITY

Fat makes food more palatable by acting as a carrier for the compounds that give food its characteristic flavours and aromas. It also imparts a certain texture and creamy mouth feel. The texture of fat is caused by the presence of small globules of fat, sized 0.1–3 μm. The creamy texture of fat can be imitated by similar sized particles of protein and starch, and this technique is used in some fat substitutes, which are increasingly being used as an ingredient in some low fat products.

■ 5.5.8 PROVISION OF THE ESSENTIAL FATTY ACIDS

The indispensable role of fat in the diet is the provision of the essential fatty acids (linoleic and α-linolenic acid and their derivatives). Linoleic acid deficiency does not arise in individuals selecting their own diets, but has been observed in infants fed on skimmed milk, in patients with chronic fat malabsorption and in those undergoing total parenteral nutrition. Linoleic acid deficiency results in a variety of abnormalities. In infants it is characterized by poor growth, increased food intake, a scaly dermatitis and impaired immune response. In adults, dermatitis is the most obvious sign. In patients with fat malabsorption, the skin symptoms are improved by the topical application of linoleic acid.

An intake of linoleic acid in the region of 1–2 per cent of the dietary energy is usually adequate to prevent clinical signs of deficiency, but higher intakes may be required if fat malabsorption is present. It has been suggested that the minimal requirement in healthy infants may be as low as 0.5 per cent of energy intake. However, this was based on observations of infants fed cow's milk formula which contained 0.5 per cent energy as linoleic acid and 0.5 per cent as α-linolenic acid. Studies in rats show that α-linolenic acid has a sparing effect on the requirement for linoleic acid. This is because both the $n-6$ and $n-3$ series can partially substitute for each other as constituents of membrane phospholipids. It is generally considered that the optimal intake for linoleic acid is in the range of 3–6 per cent of the dietary energy. It has been argued that linoleic acid decreases the plasma cholesterol raising effects of saturated fatty acids such as palmitic acid which has a threshold of around 4 per cent of the dietary energy as linoleic acid. (Hayes and Khosla – Chapter 9 for a further discussion of the relationship between dietary saturated fatty acids and plasma cholesterol.)

For many years α-linolenic acid was not regarded as a dietary essential. However it has now been established that its derivative, DHA, is the major polyunsaturated fatty acid in the human brain and retina. Experiments on rats and monkeys have shown that when the maternal diet contains adequate amounts of linoleic acid but no α-linolenic acid, the level of DHA in the brain and retina of the offspring is markedly reduced and replaced with $22:5n-6$ derived from linoleic acid. This biochemical change is accompanied by impaired visual function and learning ability and an increase in voluntary fluid intake. These effects which were observed in the infant monkeys could not be reversed in later life which suggests that there is a critical window of neural development.

In preterm infants, where rates of brain growth are high, the demand for DHA outstrips the capacity to synthesize DHA from α-linolenic acid so that small amounts of DHA need to be supplied in the diet. It was first noted that visual function was abnormal in preterm infants fed artificial formula that contained both linoleic and α-linolenic acid when compared with infants fed breast milk, which contains DHA. Adding DHA to the artificial formula corrected the abnormal visual function. It is uncertain as to whether full-term infants require DHA but human milk does contain considerable amounts. Studies have shown that infants fed formula milk have a lower proportion of DHA in their brains and retinas compared with those fed breast milk. Breastfed infants have also been found to have a higher IQ than bottle-fed infants.

It has also been argued that as breast milk contains arachidonic acid, breast milk substitutes should be fortified with both DHA and arachidonic acid. Several clinical trials are in progress to assess whether there is indeed any benefit from fortifying breast milk substitutes with these long chain polyunsaturated fatty acids. The proportion of DHA in breast milk is influenced by the maternal intakes of DHA as well as the ratio of linoleic: linolenic acid in the mother's diet. For example, the concentrations of DHA in breast milk of vegan women is only one-third of the concentration in women following an omnivorous diet (DHA is absent from vegan diets but their intakes of linoleic acid and the ratio of linoleic:linolenic acid in the diet is high).

It has been observed that a low proportion of EPA and DHA in blood lipids is associated with an increased risk of sudden cardiac death. Randomized controlled trials have also shown that an intake of about 1 g of a combination of EPA and DHA decreases the risk of sudden cardiac death in men who have already had a heart attack. Experiments conducted in animals suggest that DHA, in particular, may protect against abnormal heart rhythms (arrhythmias) that are associated with sudden cardiac death. The exact mechanism, however, remains uncertain. But the evidence is sufficiently strong to justify the recommendation that the average UK diet should supply at least 0.2 g of long chain $n-3$ fatty acid(s).

The estimated requirement for linolenic acid is about 0.2–0.5 per cent of the dietary energy intake. Both the $n-3$ and $n-6$ fatty acids are required in the diet and their intakes need to be balanced. An optimal $n-6:n-3$ ratio is estimated to be between 5:1 and 10:1.

Long chain $n-3$ fatty acids, particularly DHA, seem to protect against cardiac arrhythmias and sudden cardiac death

■ 5.5.9 ROLE OF N-3 AND N-6 FATTY ACIDS AS PHARMACOLOGICAL AGENTS

High intakes of fish oil containing eicosapentaenoic acid (EPA) and docosahexaenoic acid (DHA) display several pharmacological properties: inhibition of inflammation, antithrombotic effects, altered lipoprotein metabolism, inhibition of atherosclerosis, decreased blood pressure and inhibition of tumour growth. Fish oil preparations containing a daily dose of about 3 g of EPA/DHA are used as licensed medicines to lower plasma triacylglycerol concentrations in patients with hypertriglyceridaemia. Concentrates of EPA and DHA are also licensed for the prevention of coronary heart disease. Pharmacological preparations containing EPA and DHA have also been shown in placebo-controlled clinical trials to bring about some symptomatic relief in rheumatoid arthritis, colitis, psoriasis, Crohn's disease and systemic lupus erythematosus. They also significantly improve survival in patients with IgA nephropathy.

There is some evidence to suggest that Δ6 desaturase activity is impaired in some metabolic disorders, particularly in diabetes. It has been argued that this metabolic block could be circumvented by consuming γ-linolenic acid. Δ6 desaturase is generally not expressed in plants but there are some exceptions, e.g. the evening primrose (*Oenothera biennis*) and the starflower (*Borago officinalis*). Oils derived from these plants contain gamma-linolenic acid ($18:3n-6$) and are widely sold in health food shops with health claims that they bypass any metabolic block in the synthesis of arachidonic acid from linoleic acid and may be of value in premenstrual syndrome and eczema. It is claimed that the consumption of gamma-linolenic acid increases the production of 1-series prostaglandins from dihomogammalinolenic acid.

Conjugated linoleic acid (mainly 18:2 9-*cis*, 11 *trans*) when consumed in large amounts by rats prevents the development of cancer in individuals exposed to carcinogens. It is also claimed to promote weight loss. It is sold as a health food supplement but there is no evidence that it is of benefit to human health.

■ 5.6 RELATIONSHIP BETWEEN THE INTAKE OF POLYUNSATURATED FATTY ACIDS AND VITAMIN E INTAKE

The requirement for vitamin E is linked to the intake of polyunsaturated fatty acids. The role of vitamin E is to protect polyunsaturated fatty acids in membranes from damage by free radicals. Free radicals are formed from polyunsaturated fatty acids by the abstraction of hydrogen from a double bond usually followed by translocation of double bonds to give a conjugated double bond system, and reaction with oxygen to form lipid peroxides.

Lipid peroxidation stimulates a chain reaction generating further lipid peroxides. Lipid peroxidation leads to damage of the structure of proteins and cell membranes. The requirement for vitamin E is approximately 0.4 mg vitamin E/g polyunsaturated fatty acid. Fortunately, those vegetable oils that are rich in polyunsaturated fatty acids are good sources of vitamin E. The greater the number of double bonds in a fatty acid, the more susceptible it is to oxidation. Consequently, more vitamin E is needed to protect polyunsaturated fatty acids with five and six double bonds such as EPA and DHA. Fish oils are a poor source of vitamin E and it is well known that high intakes of fish oil in animals can induce vitamin E deficiency which can be prevented by additional intake of vitamin E. Approximately 3–4 mg vitamin E/g are needed to protect EPA and DHA.

■ 5.7 DIETARY INTAKES OF FAT

Variations in dietary fat intake between different populations are mainly due to differences in the amount of fat present in animal products (dairy and meat products) and the amount and type of fat used in food preparation.

As a general rule, as countries become more affluent they consume more fat. Intakes in rural Africa, South East Asia, India, and China are often as low as 15 per cent of the energy intake (30–40 g/day) whereas those in Australasia, North America and Europe are approximately 40 per cent of the energy intake (90–120 g/day). The globalization of food has contributed to more uniformity of fat intakes in urban areas.

Human diets vary not only in the amount of fat consumed but in the type of fatty acids provided. From about the mid-1960s in the USA, changes in the processing of oils and fats led to the increased popularity of liquid vegetable oils for cooking and easy-to-spread margarines. The popularity of these fats in turn led to a decrease in the use of butter and lard. Similar trends can be seen in Australia and somewhat later in the UK and Europe. The increased consumption of vegetable oils and soft margarine has led to an increased intake of the polyunsaturated fatty acid linoleic acid and decline in that of saturated fatty acids.

■ 5.8 DIETARY REFERENCE VALUES FOR FAT AND FATTY ACIDS

There are upper and lower limits to the desirable intake of fat. The need for fat changes throughout the life-cycle. Relatively high intakes are needed in the first two years of life but thereafter the need for fat declines. In adults, the lower limits for fat-intake (15 per cent total energy intake) are set to ensure an adequate intake of fat-soluble vitamins and essential fatty acids, and to help meet energy needs. An upper limit of 30–35 per cent energy intake is set to help decrease the risk of obesity. Limits are set on the amount of saturated (usually less than 10 per cent energy) and *trans* fatty acids (less than 2 per cent energy) present in the diet as high intakes of these fatty acids have been linked to an increased risk of cardiovascular disease. An intake of 6 per cent energy as polyunsaturated fatty acids is recommended (5 per cent energy from linoleic acid and 1 per cent from α-linolenic acid and long chain $n-3$ fatty acids). An upper limit to the intake of polyunsaturated fatty acids is set at 10 per cent of the energy because of uncertainties regarding the long-term effects of higher intakes.

SUMMARY

- Fat consist of fatty acids and esters of fatty acids.
- Dietary fat and adipose tissue consist mainly of triacylglycerols which are used to supply and store energy.
- Fat supplies and facilitates the absorption of fat-soluble vitamins.
- Two series of essential fatty acids required by humans (the *n-6* derived from linoleic and the *n-3* derived from α-linolenic acid) are both needed as constituents of membrane phospholipids.
- Linoleic acid has a specific role in maintaining the permeability barrier of the skin and gives rise to arachidonic acid which is the major eicosanoid precursor.
- Docosahexaenoic acid is a major constituent of brain and retinal phospholipids.

FURTHER READING

Christie, W.W. *What is a lipid*? Online. Available at www.lipid.co.uk (accessed 23rd September 2002).

British Nutrition Foundation Task Force on Unsaturated Fatty Acids (1994). London: Chapman Hall.

Elia, M. and Livesey, G. (1992) 'Energy expenditure and fuel selection in biological systems: the theory and practice of calculations based on indirect calorimetry and tracer methods', *World Review of Nutrition and Dietetics*, 70: 68–131.

Gurr, M.L., Harwood, J.L. and Frayn, K.N. (2002) *Lipid Biochemistry*, 5th edn, Oxford: Blackwell.

Hayes, K.C. and Khosla, P. (1992) 'Dietary fatty acid thresholds and cholesterolemia' *FASEB* J., 6(8): 2600–7.

Sanders, T.A.B. (1999) 'Essential fatty acid requirements of vegetarians in pregnancy, lactation, and infancy', *Am. J. Clin. Nutr*, 70: 555S–559S.

6 MINERALS

The body contains a number of inorganic elements in addition to the water, fat and protein which are its major components. These elements must all be supplied in the diet. The amounts required range from grams per day in the case of sodium, potassium and chloride to a few micrograms per day in the case of the trace elements such as selenium and chromium. Since they are all present in most organisms, normal varied diets are unlikely to be deficient in any of them. Occasionally deficiencies do arise in people whose food supply is restricted to plants grown in a specific geographical location where the soil lacks a particular mineral. Endemic goitre, arising from iodine deficiency, is the most common example of this in humans, although examples in animals are much more common. More recently mineral deficiencies have been observed in patients who have been maintained for a long time on total parenteral nutrition, since this requires the deliberate inclusion of purified sources of all essential nutrients. Other cases of mineral deficiencies are more likely to arise from a failure to absorb adequate quantities in the gut, or from excessive losses. Problems of mineral nutrition can also arise from toxicity, caused either by excessive consumption or by a failure to excrete the mineral in adequate amounts (see Chapter 8).

Mineral deficiencies can arise from low intake, inadequate absorption or excessive loss

■ 6.1 SODIUM, POTASSIUM AND CHLORIDE

These monovalent electrolytes are the major solutes in body fluids, and are thus responsible for the osmolarity and volume of both the intra- and the extracellular fluid (ICF and ECF). Hence the balance of these minerals within the body is intimately linked with water balance. Their other functions include conduction of electrical signals in nerves and excitation of muscle, and the consequences of deficiencies or excesses often affect the functioning of the heart or the skeletal muscles. These electrolytes are also responsible, in combination with the bicarbonate system, for regulating the pH of the body, and deficiencies and excesses may be associated with alterations in acid-base balance. Sodium and chloride are also linked to the transport of many small molecules across cell membranes, and their presence is necessary for the absorption of several nutrients from the gut.

Deficiencies or excesses of sodium, potassium or chloride are rare. However, there is considerable epidemiological evidence showing an association between high intakes of sodium, low intakes of potassium and the prevalence of essential hypertension (high blood pressure) in a population. This evidence is supported by studies showing that decreasing sodium intake or increasing potassium intake in hypertensive subjects reduces their blood pressure. However, the exact mechanisms by which these effects are mediated is not entirely clear (see Chapter 9).

Sodium deficiency is rare, but high intake of sodium chloride may be a cause of high blood pressure

A 70 kg body contains about 3.5 mol sodium, 3.2 mol potassium and 2.1 mol chloride. Half the sodium is in the ECF, where it accounts for 95 per cent of the cations, and only 10 per cent is intracellular. The rest is in bone, where it is not fully exchangeable with the ECF. In contrast more than 90 per cent of potassium is exchangeable, and most of it is in the ICF, where it accounts for 85 per cent of the cations, with only about 80 mmol in the ECF. The distribution of sodium and potassium is maintained by the Na^+/K^+-linked ATPase enzymes present on all cell membranes. Chloride is like sodium in being predominantly extracellular, although all of it is exchangeable. The major intracellular anion is phosphate.

■ 6.1.1 SODIUM INTAKE

The intake of sodium varies widely within a population, and even more widely between different populations. In the UK the average intake is around 150 mmol/d (3.5 g Na^+, equivalent to 9 g NaCl), with 90 per cent of individual intakes falling within the range 60–260 mmol/d). More than 90 per cent of sodium is consumed as sodium chloride, which is present naturally in many foods of animal origin and which is also added to many foods as a preservative and for flavouring. Other sodium salts are also added to foods for specific purposes, including bicarbonate in baking powder, sulphite and propionate as preservatives, and monosodium glutamate as a flavour enhancer. More than 80 per cent of sodium intake comes from processed foods.

Most dietary sodium comes from processed foods

Bread alone accounts for one quarter of the sodium in the average UK diet. Savoury foods such as bacon, ham and cheese are also significant sources of sodium because salt has been used to preserve them. Sodium intakes have fallen over the past fifty years because of changes in methods of food preparation and the decline in bread intake. However, much of the sodium intake nowadays comes from ready-prepared meals. The use of food composition tables and diet records is not a reliable way to estimate sodium intake. This is because processed foods contain varying amounts of salt but also because salt can be added during cooking or at the table, which together are known as discretionary sources of sodium. These discretionary sources only account for about 15 per cent of sodium intake on average, but they account for a much greater proportion of the intake of those who consume the greatest amounts of sodium.

■ 6.1.2 SODIUM EXCRETION

Absorption of sodium from the gut is normally virtually complete, and although some sodium is secreted into the gut in bile, pancreatic juice and small intestinal secretions, no more than 2 per cent of excretion is via the faeces. Another 2 per cent is via the skin, although more can be lost this way if there is active sweating. People who are acclimatized to hot climates produce a more dilute sweat to avoid excessive loss of sodium. Thus more than 95 per cent of sodium is excreted in the urine, and since most people are in sodium balance the urinary excretion of sodium is generally taken to be the most reliable way of estimating sodium intake.

The healthy adult kidney is able to excrete as much or as little sodium as required, as long as there is sufficient water. However it cannot concentrate the urine above a specific gravity of 1.035 g/ml; this is why shipwrecked sailors should not drink sea-water because there will be insufficient water to excrete all the sodium. At the other extreme sodium balance can be maintained on intakes down to 10 mmol/d (about 0.6 g sodium chloride).

Urinary sodium excretion depends on the balance between glomerular filtration and tubular reabsorption, and these are sensitive to changes in ECF volume and blood pressure. Several mechanisms, both neural and hormonal, appear to be involved in this regulation, including the renin/angiotensin/aldosterone system and an atrial natriuretic peptide (see Box 6.1). Deficient and excessive amounts of sodium in the body can occur

Sodium balance can be maintained over a wide range of intakes

---

BOX 6.1 CONTROL OF SODIUM BALANCE BY THE RENIN/ANGIOTENSIN/ ALDOSTERONE SYSTEM

In response to a decrease in extracellular fluid volume or low sodium concentration, the kidney secretes the enzyme renin, which catalyses the conversion of the globulin angiotensinogen (made in the liver) to angiotensin I. In the vessels of the lungs this is modified to angiotensin II by the angiotensin converting enzyme (ACE). This in turn acts on the adrenal cortex to cause secretion of the mineralocorticoid aldosterone, which increases reabsorption of sodium in the renal tubules. Ultimately, as sodium is retained, this causes secretion of anti-diuretic hormone, and thus fluid is retained, thus returning the extracellular fluid volume and composition to normal. These actions are opposed by atrial natriuretic peptide, a hormone which is secreted by the heart in response to increased blood pressure and volume and which promotes the excretion of sodium and water by the kidneys.

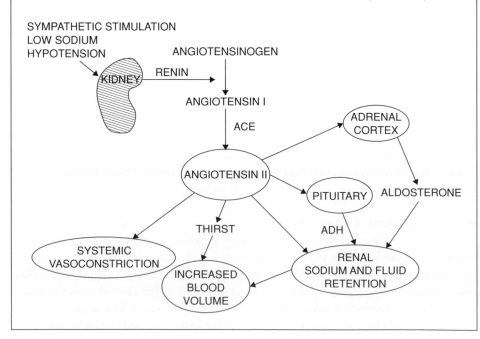

as a result of excessive or inadequate excretion of sodium. For example in Addison's disease the adrenal cortex is impaired, resulting in hyposecretion of aldosterone and hence failure to reabsorb adequate amounts of sodium. Excessive amounts of sodium can also be lost through prolonged heavy vomiting and diarrhoea, or from regular heavy intermittent bouts of sweating, as in the case of so-called miners cramps. The consequences of sodium depletion include muscle weakness, cramps and wasting, taste abnormalities and unpredictable swings in fluid balance. They are graphically described by McCance (1936), who induced sodium depletion in human volunteers by a combination of low sodium intake and frequent sessions of heat-induced sweating.

Sodium retention, leading to oedema, can occur in chronic renal failure, in heart failure, or through excessive aldosterone secretion from a tumour of the adrenal cortex. One of the consequences of sodium retention is an increase in blood pressure. However in the vast majority of patients with high blood pressure, the concentration of sodium in the plasma and extracellular fluid is normal. Nevertheless, restricting the intake of sodium chloride is effective in lowering blood pressure and diuretic drugs which are used to treat high blood pressure are effective in promoting sodium excretion.

The immature kidneys of young infants who are fed on unmodified cow's milk may also be unable to excrete enough sodium, particularly if insufficient water is given to drink, since cow's milk contains five times as much sodium as human breast milk. The infant develops hypernatraemia, and may show such symptoms as diarrhoea, skin rash and, in extreme cases, convulsions. Hence modern infant formulae are all modified to reduce the solute load.

■ 6.1.3 POTASSIUM BALANCE

Values for potassium intake vary over a smaller range than those for sodium intake, averaging approximately 70 mmol/d in the UK. Fruit and vegetables, especially bananas, are rich sources, as are meat, milk and whole grain cereals. Only one third of intake comes from processed foods.

About 10 per cent of potassium excretion is via the faeces. This is largely because in the colon sodium is reabsorbed and replaced by potassium. Cutaneous losses of potassium are minimal, so that again urine is the major route of excretion. The range over which the kidney can maintain potassium balance is not quite as extensive as that for sodium, with negative balances being reported on intakes below 25 mmol/d. Although most filtered potassium is reabsorbed in the proximal tubule, aldosterone acts on the distal tubule to promote the secretion of potassium alongside the reabsorption of sodium.

Potassium depletion can occur if losses are excessive. Thiazide diuretics and synthetic steroids both cause increased urinary excretion of potassium; excessive vomiting and diarrhoea can also cause potassium depletion. The consequences of potassium depletion are muscle weakness, mental confusion and increased cardiac excitability. Potassium excess is less common, but can occur as a consequence of renal failure. However it is potentially more serious, since it may lead to cardiac arrest.

Because only 2 per cent of the potassium in the body is extracellular, measurements of plasma potassium concentrations are not a very reliable guide to potassium status. On the other hand, if whole body potassium content can be measured it does provide a good estimate of lean body mass, since most of the potassium is concentrated within the cells of the lean tissue. Potassium can be measured by monitoring gamma radiation from the isotope ^{40}K, which occurs naturally as 0.012 per cent of potassium and has a half-life of 1,300 million years. Thus the whole body gamma counter has become a useful research tool for measuring changes in body composition. Loss of lean tissue as a consequence of nutritional depletion results in loss of potassium, and this needs to be replaced during nutritional rehabilitation. Potassium intakes like those of sodium can be assessed indirectly by measuring potassium excretion in urine.

Potassium is a good marker of body cell mass

■ 6.1.4 CHLORIDE BALANCE

Most chloride is consumed as sodium chloride, so total chloride intake is slightly lower than total sodium intake. Urine is also the route by which most chloride is excreted, with molar ratios of sodium to chloride usually very close to unity. Chloride is actively reabsorbed in the distal tubule and the large intestine, and replaced by secreted bicarbonate. Deficiencies and excesses of chloride usually accompany those of sodium, though occasionally pure chloride depletion is seen following excessive loss of gastric hydrochloric acid from pyloric stenosis or self-induced vomiting. There is some evidence that high intakes of sodium chloride play a role in the development of high blood pressure, and that this is the reason for the epidemiological association between high intakes of salt and the incidence of hypertension. A high intake of sodium chloride increases blood pressure in susceptible individuals but neither potassium chloride nor sodium bicarbonate have this effect.

■ 6.2 CALCIUM, PHOSPHORUS, MAGNESIUM AND FLUORIDE

These minerals are all found mainly in the skeleton where they form the rigid mineral support which the body requires. However, the small proportions of each which exist as soluble ions within and around cells also have very important functions.

■ 6.2.1 FUNCTIONS OF CALCIUM

The adult skeleton contains about 1 kg calcium in a complex crystalline material known as hydroxyapatite. This is deposited on an organic matrix of collagen by cells known as osteoblasts. These are active throughout life, as are osteoclasts, which are responsible for resorption of bone. For about the first thirty years of life there is net deposition of calcium in bone at a rate of up to 150 mg/d in infants and children and up to 300 mg/d in adolescents. The most rapid accretion of calcium is between the ages of 12–13 years in girls and between 14–15 years in boys and calcium intake in this critical period determines peak bone mass. However after about the age of thirty, when peak bone mass has been reached, osteoclast activity predominates resulting in a net loss of bone mineral. Although the need for calcium for bone growth is clearly the major factor determining the requirement for calcium in infants and children, there is no simple relationship between the amount of calcium consumed and the rate of bone mineral deposition during growth or bone mineral loss during later life. However, recent research suggests that high calcium intakes during the period of rapid bone calcification in adolescents can improve bone density.

The rate at which bone mineral is lost in later life appears to be a constant fraction of peak bone mass, although there is usually an acceleration in females at or after the menopause. This can lead to a condition known as osteoporosis, in which the amount of bone per unit volume is decreased but the composition of the bone remains unchanged. The bone structure becomes porous, because of the removal of mineral by the osteoblasts, leaving the bone weak and liable to fracture. Osteoporosis is clinically important because it leads to a high incidence of crush fractures of the vertebrae and fractures of the neck or femur, both of which lead to pain and disability and further morbidity and mortality.

Failure of the bone to become properly mineralized during growth leads to the disease rickets in children and osteomalacia in adults. This is characterized by skeletal deformities, bone pain and muscle weakness. However, like osteoporosis, rickets and osteomalacia are not simply caused by a low intake of calcium; rather, the cause of rickets and osteomalacia is deficiency of vitamin D, which may arise from either nutritional or metabolic causes.

About 1 per cent of the body's calcium is outside the skeleton. It is present in the plasma at a concentration of 2.2–2.6 mM, of which 50 per cent is ionized. Calcium ions are required for activation of the coagulation cascade which culminates in the generation of insoluble fibrin from soluble fibrinogen. The clotting cascade consists of a series of serine proteases that exist in inactive (zymogen) and active (protease) forms. The divalent calcium ions are necessary for the activation of these clotting factors and also help stabilize the prothrombinase complex which converts fibrinogen to fibrin. Calcium ions form a bridge between the vitamin K-dependent clotting factors VII, VIII, IX, X and prothrombin and platelet membranes. The calcium binds to gamma-carboxyglutamic acid (GLA) residues in these clotting proteins and forms a bridge with the negatively charged phospholipid in the platelet membrane; this then causes a conformational change in the protein. The calcium ions suck the negatively charged GLA residue into the protein interior and force the hydrophobic residues towards the outside which bury themselves into the phospholipids bilayer of the platelet membrane. Calcium is also required within cells as an activator of phosphorylases and phosphatases, which in turn regulate many other enzymes, so that calcium is often considered as a 'second messenger'. It is also necessary for the release of several hormones and hormone releasing factors. Various channel mechanisms exist that lead to a large, transient increase in the intracellular Ca^{2+} concentration, thereby triggering a physiological event, such as the phosphoinositide (PI) cascade. In the PI cascade, inositol 1,4,5-triphosphate (IP3) is released from the plasma membrane into the cytosol where it causes the rapid release of Ca^{2+} from intracellular stores. This induces calmodulin to bind 3 or 4 Ca^{2+} ions. In its bound state, calmodulin can activate many enzymes and transporters.

Calcium is particularly important in muscles, including the heart, since it is involved in excitation contraction coupling. The arrival of an action potential at the muscle cell membrane causes release of calcium from the sarcoplasmic reticulum into the cytosol of the muscle fibre where it stimulates the myofibrillar ATPase, causing the myofibril to contract. It is also involved in synaptic transmission.

■ 6.2.2 CALCIUM BALANCE

Calcium balance can be maintained over a wide range of intakes: 95 per cent of adults in the UK consume between 260 and 1,300 mg/d from food, but higher and lower values are recorded in other countries without apparent ill effect. The main dietary sources are

Calcium balance can
be maintained over a
wide range of intakes

milk and milk products, contributing 50 per cent, with cereal products contributing another 25 per cent largely because flour is fortified with calcium carbonate. In addition hard water can contribute another 200 mg per day.

Most absorption of calcium occurs in the jejunum, though some is also absorbed in the ileum and the colon. The main route of excretion is the faeces. This represents not only unabsorbed dietary calcium but also calcium secreted in the bile and pancreatic juice and desquamated cells. Some calcium is also excreted in the urine, although 97 per cent of filtered calcium is reabsorbed in the tubules. Urinary calcium excretion appears to rise on high protein and sodium intakes, but this does seem to affect calcium balance significantly in the short term. However, in the longer term it may contribute to osteo-porosis. Conditions that result in metabolic acidosis such as alcoholism also increase the rate of loss of calcium from bones.

A number of mechanisms are involved in maintaining calcium balance, the most important endocrine factors being vitamin D, parathyroid hormone and calcitonin (see Figure 6.2). The main targets of these systems are the gut, where calcium absorption is controlled, the kidney, where renal excretion is controlled, and bone, where the balance between calcium mobilization and deposition is controlled. The result of these interactions is to maintain plasma calcium concentration within narrow limits while at the same time ensuring that calcium is deposited in the bone during growth; calcium is transferred to the foetus during pregnancy and is secreted in the milk during lactation. Dairy cows occasionally fail to adapt rapidly enough to the massive increase in calcium output in the milk at the beginning of lactation, and this can cause hypocalcaemia in the condition known as 'milk fever'.

The active metabolite of vitamin D (1, 25-dihydroxycholecalciferol) is now considered as a hormone involved in regulating calcium homeostasis. This stimulates calcium trans-port across the cells of the small intestine by promoting the synthesis of a calcium-binding protein within the villus cells, resulting in increased absorption of dietary calcium. It also acts on both osteoblasts and osteoclasts to mobilize calcium. The osteoblasts produce cytokines which act locally to stimulate osteoclast activity, while the formation of new osteoclasts is also promoted.

Vitamin D is a major
dietary factor affecting
calcium balance

Parathyroid hormone acts on the kidney both to promote reabsorption of calcium and to stimulate the activity of the 1-alpha hydroxylase enzyme, thereby activating vitamin D, which promotes calcium absorption from the gut. Parathyroid hormone also acts on osteoblasts to promote resorption of calcium from bone.

• **Figure 6.2** The role of parathyroid hormone and vitamin D in calcium balance

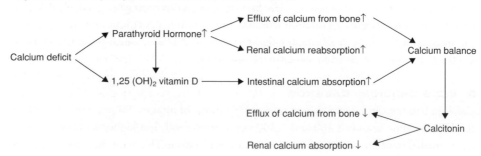

Calcitonin is secreted by the thyroid gland in response to increasing plasma calcium concentration. It acts to restore plasma calcium homeostasis by inhibiting osteoclast activity and inhibiting the reabsorption of calcium in the renal tubule. In practice, it only makes a small contribution to regulating calcium balance.

■ 6.2.3 PHOSPHORUS

The body contains almost as much phosphorus as calcium, and the metabolism of the two minerals is intimately connected. However, only 85 per cent of phosphorus is present in bone, as phosphate ions in the crystalline structure of hydroxyapatite. The rest is distributed throughout the body, but again as phosphate groups. Phosphate is part of the structure of nucleic acids, and of many proteins, carbohydrates and phospholipids as well as small molecules such as ATP and creatine phosphate. Phosphate groups on the surface of many of these molecules carry charges, allowing them to interact in more hydrophilic areas of the cell. Phosphorylation and dephosphorylation are also very common ways of activating or suppressing enzymes for the purpose of metabolic control. The energy stored in the high energy bond of ATP and creatine phosphate allows energy to be transferred between different metabolic reactions, and to fuel the contraction of actomyosin.

Because of its wide distribution in plant and animal cells, phosphorus is present in most foodstuffs. The average intake in the UK is 1.2 g/d. About 60 per cent is absorbed in the small intestine, and this proportion falls when there is vitamin D deficiency. Some of the phosphorus present in plant foods, notably legumes and whole grain cereals, is in the form of phytic acid (inositol hexaphosphate) which forms insoluble complexes with divalent cations such as calcium, magnesium, zinc and iron, thereby inhibiting their absorption from the gut. Plasma phosphate concentration appears to be regulated mainly by urinary excretion. Parathyroid hormone and calcitonin both increase phosphate excretion.

Most human diets contain roughly equal amounts of calcium and phosphorus, and this allows normal growth and homeostasis. However, the diets of some farm animals can be less well balanced, with forages tending to be lacking in phosphate while some of the concentrates fed to highly productive cattle are low in calcium. Such imbalances can lead to excessive excretion of both minerals and they ultimately produce signs of rickets or osteomalacia.

■ 6.2.4 MAGNESIUM

About 70 per cent of the body's 25 g of magnesium is in bone, where magnesium ions are closely associated with hydroxyl ions in the crystal structure. Most of the rest is within the cells of all soft tissues, where it is a cofactor in numerous reactions, particularly those involved in energy metabolism, as well as DNA replication and RNA synthesis. One per cent of magnesium is in the extracellular fluid, where it is required to maintain a stable electrical gradient across the membranes of nerves, muscles and the heart. Hence magnesium deficiency leads to muscle weakness, tetany, tachycardia and ventricular fibrillation. Magnesium is also involved in the release of parathyroid hormone, so that hypomagnesaemia is often accompanied by hypocalcaemia.

Magnesium is equally abundant in plant cells, particularly in the chloroplasts of green plants, so that most foodstuffs contribute to magnesium intake. One-third of the intake in the UK is derived from cereals, with another 20 per cent from green vegetables. The average intake is 280 mg/d, and absorption in the small intestine is normally very efficient.

Magnesium is excreted mainly in the urine, and this process responds rapidly to changes in intake to maintain homeostasis. Magnesium balance can certainly be maintained on intakes of 50 mg/d, with evidence of adaptation to much lower intakes, so deficiencies and excesses are rare. Hypomagnesaemia in humans only occurs as a result of starvation, malabsorption, excessive vomiting and diarrhoea or excessive urinary loss because of renal disease or drug ingestion. In cattle, acute hypomagnesaemia sometimes occurs when they are turned out to low magnesium grassland after a winter of high concentrate feeding, and this results in tetany being known as "grass staggers".

■ 6.2.5 FLUORIDE

At least 99 per cent of fluoride in the body is present in the bones and teeth, at a concentration which varies with the amount of fluoride ingested. Fluoride ions can partially replace hydroxyl ions, producing a stronger structure and promoting remineralization. However, excessive accumulation produces the toxic signs of fluorosis. Mild fluorosis, which can occur in a small proportion of sensitive children on intakes as low as 1 ppm in the water, is characterized by mottling of the teeth. This involves yellow or brown staining and pitting of the enamel, which is weak and wears rapidly. More severe fluorosis, typically on intakes above 10 ppm, produces outgrowths of the bone, thickening of joints and calcification of tendons, causing stiffness, deformity and lameness.

In contrast, soft tissues do not accumulate fluoride, and it has no known functions there. Indeed there is no direct evidence that fluoride is essential in humans, although this may be partly because it is very difficult to produce a totally fluoride-free diet. However, impaired growth and fertility in experimental animals fed on highly purified diets has been shown to respond to the inclusion of 1–2 ppm fluoride.

The only rich dietary sources of fluoride are fish and tea, and most of the fluoride we consume comes from drinking water. Average intakes in the UK are 1–2 mg per day, but there is considerable variation. Soluble fluoride is very efficiently absorbed, mainly from the stomach, and excretion is mainly via the urine.

The fluoride content of water varies widely in different geographical locations, and it has been observed that the incidence of dental caries varies inversely with the fluoride content of the water. There have now been numerous studies showing that fluoridation of water up to a level of 1 ppm always decreases the incidence of dental caries and never increases the incidence of any other disease. Nevertheless only about 10 per cent of people in the UK have the benefit of fluoridated water, although fluoride-containing toothpaste is now widely available and this does appear to have decreased the incidence of dental caries in recent decades (the role of fluoride in dental caries is further discussed in Chapter 9).

Fluoridation of water is a very effective way of preventing dental caries

■ 6.3 IRON, COPPER AND ZINC

These are all transition metals which act as prosthetic groups in a large number of enzymes. In many cases their function depends on their ability to switch between redox states, so that they catalyse oxidation and reduction reactions, including defence against free radical damage. However, this property also means that potentially they could catalyse undesirable oxidative damage, so that the concentrations of free metal ions is carefully controlled.

■ 6.3.1 FUNCTIONS OF IRON

More than half the iron in the body is present in the red blood cells as haemoglobin, with the function of carrying oxygen around the body. Each molecule of haemoglobin consists of four protein chains and four haem groups. The iron atom at the centre of the haem group is attached to four nitrogen atoms within the haem group and one histidine residue in the protein, leaving one site vacant to bind with oxygen. This allows the haemoglobin to become saturated with oxygen in the lungs, and for some of the oxygen to dissociate from the haemoglobin as it passes through the other tissues, according to their requirement.

Myoglobin is a protein which binds oxygen in muscle, to act as a temporary store. Its structure is similar to haemoglobin, but with only one haem group and one protein chain per molecule. Cytochromes have a similar composition, but different structures, and only that of cytochrome c allows it to bind to oxygen. Thus the other cytochromes function to transfer reducing equivalents in the form of electrons, particularly in the mitochondrial electron transport chain which generates ATP. There are also many other iron-containing enzymes with a wide variety of functions.

Iron is stored in the body, but in order to avoid adverse effects it is stored in the interior of a protein, ferritin. Most ferritin is in the liver, with small amounts in plasma and other tissues. Some iron is also stored in haemosiderin, which contains some ferritin-like protein but also some colloidal ferric hydroxide. Iron is transported between different compartments of the body bound to the protein transferrin.

The clearest effect of iron deficiency is an impaired capacity for exercise and work, because the oxidative capacity of muscle is reduced. In severe anaemia this would be exacerbated by reduced oxygen delivery. There is also evidence of impairment of a number of functions of the brain in iron deficiency. Several parts of the brain have a relatively high iron content, and this increases during the first three decades of life. However, the extent to which chronic iron deficiency actually impairs the development of cognitive and intellectual function is still not defined. Similarly, although there is evidence that immunological function is impaired in iron deficiency, there are no good data showing a greater incidence or severity of infectious diseases attributable solely to iron deficiency.

■ 6.3.2 IRON METABOLISM

In the UK, about 20 per cent of iron is derived from meat and meat products, in the form of haem iron, while over 40 per cent is derived from cereal products including bread, which is fortified with iron by law. Haem iron is relatively well absorbed (about 25 per cent) in the small intestine, whereas inorganic or non-haem iron is absorbed much less efficiently, typically only around 5 per cent. Inorganic iron can only be absorbed in the reduced (Fe^{2+}) form, so its absorption is enhanced by the presence of reducing agents such as ascorbic acid. On the other hand there are a number of substances which impair iron absorption, including dietary fibre, phytate and tannins, which all form insoluble complexes in the gut. Acid conditions also favour iron absorption, and gastric acid forms

Iron in the haem form from animal products is much better absorbed than iron from plant sources

soluble complexes with iron which remain soluble at the higher pH of the small intestine. Thus a lack of gastric acid diminishes iron absorption.

Once inside the mucosal cell the porphyrin ring of haem is split, releasing the iron to mix with the pool of inorganic iron which binds to ferritin. Iron can only move out of the mucosa and into the circulation if it can bind to transferrin. This allows some regulation of iron absorption in relation to body iron status. If the body is replete, transferrin will be saturated and any iron which enters the mucosa will be lost back into the lumen of the gut, whereas if transferrin saturation is low the efficiency of absorption of iron will increase. Unfortunately this also means that absorption of a single large dose of iron, such as a therapeutic supplement, tends to inhibit iron uptake for several subsequent days, so that supplements need to be taken less frequently to be absorbed more efficiently.

Iron is transported to the bone marrow, where it is used for the synthesis of haemoglobin. Red blood cells have a lifetime of about 120 days, after which they are taken up by macrophages of the reticulo-endothelial system, where the iron is released and passed to transferrin in the plasma for recirculation. Little iron is excreted in the urine, and basal losses consist mostly of the turnover of cells from the skin, the intestines, the urinary tract and the airways. However iron is also lost whenever blood is lost, and thus in women of reproductive age there is a regular loss of iron in menstrual blood. This amounts to an average of 0.56 mg/d, averaged over the whole cycle, in addition to basal losses of 0.8 mg/d.

In spite of the body's efficiency in re-utilizing iron, iron deficiency is extremely common. In industrialized countries 10–15 per cent of women have menstrual losses which are heavier than can be met from their normal diet, and in developing countries, where the intake of haem iron is lower, the proportion is greater. In many tropical countries infestation with intestinal parasites such as hookworm causes further blood loss which puts many more people at risk from iron deficiency.

■ 6.3.3 ASSESSMENT OF IRON STATUS

When iron status is inadequate haemoglobin production will be impaired. This will gradually lead to the development of anaemia, which means a low concentration of haemoglobin in the blood. The anaemia will be of the microcytic, hypochromic type, meaning that the erythrocytes are smaller than normal (decreased mean corpuscular volume, MCV) and each cell contains less haemoglobin (decreased mean corpuscular haemoglobin concentration, MCHC). However, it will take some time before the haemoglobin concentration is low enough to be defined as anaemia, which is usually taken as below the 2.5th centile of the population.

Anaemia is a manifestation of quite severe iron deficiency

It is thus useful to employ more sensitive measures of iron status. The first measurable effect of iron deficiency is a decrease in iron stores, and this is reflected in a decrease in plasma ferritin concentration. Serum ferritin is usually below 15 μg/l by the time no stainable iron can be found in bone marrow smears. At the same time the saturation of transferrin in the plasma decreases, and when it falls below 16 per cent no more iron is delivered to red blood cell precursors.

■ 6.3.4 FUNCTIONS OF COPPER

More than 60 per cent of the copper in plasma is bound to the protein caeruloplasmin, which was previously thought to be simply a transport protein but now appears to function

• **Figure 6.3** Functions of copper-containing enzymes

Caeruloplasmin

$Fe^{2+} \rightarrow Fe^{3+}$

Cytochrome c oxidase

reduced cytochrome c + ADP + P_i + $^1/_2$ O_2 → oxidized cytochrome c + ATP + H_2O

Lysyl oxidase

lysine residue in elastin   →   allysine residue in elastin

Tyrosinase

tyrosine → DOPA (dihydroxyphenylalanine) → DOPAquinone

Dopamine-β-hydroxylase

dopamine + ascorbate + O_2 → noradrenaline + dehydroascorbate + H_2O

Superoxide dismutase

$O_2^- + O_2^- + 2H^+ \rightarrow O_2 + H_2O_2$

as a ferroxidase enzyme. Thus iron crosses cell membranes in the ferrous (Fe^{2+}) form and is then oxidized by caeruloplasmin to the ferric (Fe^{3+}) form in order to bind to the transport protein transferrin. Thus copper deficiency causes a hypochromic anaemia, and some cases of iron deficiency anaemia respond more rapidly to supplementation with a mixture of copper and iron salts than with iron alone.

Other redox enzymes containing copper include cytochrome oxidase, the terminal oxidase in the respiratory chain, which renders the nervous system, with its high energy requirement, vulnerable to copper deficiency. The nervous system is also affected by the activity of the copper-dependent enzyme dopamine β-hydroxylase in the synthesis of noradrenaline. Hence lambs with the copper deficiency "swayback" exhibit ataxia. Superoxide dismutase, an intracellular antioxidant enzyme which protects the cell from free radical damage, also contains copper.

One feature of copper deficiency in many species is weakness of connective tissue. This appears to be due to the role of copper in the enzyme lysyl oxidase, which oxidizes some of the ε-amino groups of lysine residues in proteins such as elastin to allysine, which then condenses with other allysine residues to form desmosine links, providing a strong, elastic tertiary structure. Thus children with the inherited copper deficiency disease known as Menkes syndrome usually die when their aorta ruptures. Copper is also required in the formation of disulphide cross-links in keratin, so that the hair of copper-deficient subjects develops a characteristic steely texture. The hair also lacks pigment because of the role of copper in the enzyme tyrosinase, which is involved in the synthesis of the pigment melanin.

■ 6.3.5 COPPER METABOLISM

Copper is present in a wide range of foods, though there are few important rich sources. Previously some was also obtained from contamination by copper water pipes and cooking vessels, particularly where the water was soft (acidic). Milk is rather a poor source of copper, and copper deficiency has been seen in premature infants born with low copper reserves and fed for prolonged periods on milk-based formulae, and also in malnourished children who have lost copper in repeated episodes of diarrhoea and are rehabilitated on milk-based diets.

Copper is absorbed from the small intestine, and net absorption varies inversely with copper status of the body. This may be mediated by induction of the protein metallothionein in the cells of the intestinal epithelium. Metallothionein binds both copper and zinc, and inhibits their uptake into the body. Both zinc and iron block the uptake of copper, and copper deficiency has been seen as a consequence of excessive zinc supplementation. Net absorption may also be regulated by the amount of copper secreted into the bile, since this is poorly reabsorbed and represents the major route of excretion. Copper status is usually assessed from measurements of serum or plasma copper concentration.

■ 6.3.6 FUNCTIONS OF ZINC

Zinc is a cofactor for over a hundred different enzymes in all branches of metabolism including superoxide dismutase, lactate dehydrogenase, alcohol dehydrogenase, aldolase, carbonic anhydrase, alkaline phosphatase, carboxypeptidase, RNA polymerase and DNA polymerase. In many of these it is present at the active site, acting as an electron acceptor. In others, including many transcription factors which regulate gene expression, it stabilizes the protein structure, particularly in the so-called zinc finger regions. Zinc is also involved in receptor proteins for steroid and thyroid hormones and vitamins A and D, mediating their interaction with promoter regions of DNA to initiate gene transcription. Zinc stabilizes the structure of insulin stored in the pancreas, and may also stabilize some membrane structures. Zinc also appears to have a number of functions within the immune system.

Both copper and zinc are cofactors for a large number of enzymes

With such a wide variety of functions it is not surprising that zinc deficiency appears to have a number of different effects. Acute zinc deficiency is caused by an inherited defect in zinc absorption called acrodermatitis enteropathica. This is characterized by a skin rash around the mouth and nose, diarrhoea, hair loss and irritability as well as failure to thrive and susceptibility to infections. More chronic and less severe zinc deficiency, which is usually found in association with inadequate intakes of other nutrients, is associated with growth retardation, delayed sexual development, poor wound healing and loss of taste sensitivity. Zinc deficiency in humans was first reported in remote parts of Iran where the diet was particularly high in unleavened bread which is rich in phytate. In pigs zinc deficiency causes hardening and cracking of the skin known as parakeratosis. More recently, it has been argued that marginal intakes of zinc may impair immune function and trials of zinc supplementation of children in developing countries have shown zinc supplementation helps malnourished children recover more quickly from diarrhoea.

■ 6.3.7 ZINC METABOLISM

The body contains about half as much zinc as iron, i.e. about 2 g. Sixty per cent of this is in muscle and 30 per cent in bone, with the rest in all the other tissues. Less than 0.1 per cent is in plasma, making this an unreliable way of assessing zinc status. Leucocyte zinc content is probably a better measure of zinc status, but even this is not very sensitive to mild deficiency.

Meat is the major dietary source of zinc, accounting for 30 per cent of intake in the UK, with milk and cheese providing another 25 per cent. Fruit and vegetables are poor sources. Whole grain cereals are good sources, but much is lost during milling. On the other hand milling also removes fibre and phytate, both of which inhibit zinc absorption. Iron and copper also inhibit zinc absorption by competing for uptake, whereas protein, histidine, cysteine and some organic acids may increase the solubility of zinc and increase its uptake.

Small amounts of zinc are lost in the urine and sweat, with faeces representing the major route of excretion. Zinc is actively secreted into the gut, and this acts as an important mechanism for maintaining zinc homeostasis in response to changes in intake.

■ 6.4 SELENIUM, IODINE AND CHROMIUM

In contrast to the wide range of functions of many minerals the physiological role of each of these three trace elements is confined to one or two specific molecules in the body.

■ 6.4.1 SELENIUM

Selenium derives its name from the goddess of the moon (Selene) and has its place above tellurium (which means earth) in the periodic table in the same group as sulphur. Indeed it has chemical properties similar to those of sulphur, and when it is abundant it can replace some of the sulphur in the amino acids cysteine and methionine. The geological distribution of selenium is very uneven, so that in some parts of the world selenium deficiency in grazing animals is relatively common, whereas in other parts of the world selenium toxicity is a major problem. In humans, selenocysteine residues are required at the active sites of at least 12 enzymes and proteins that contain selenocystein but the two most important of these are glutathione peroxidase and thyroxine 5′-deiodinase. These are probably synthesized by post-translational modification with inorganic selenite.

Glutathione peroxidase is an intracellular, cytosolic enzyme that reduces a variety of free radicals, particularly organic peroxides, which would otherwise cause oxidative damage. It is thus part of the body's antioxidant defence system, in conjunction with vitamin E. Deficiency of selenium and vitamin E causes degeneration of cardiac and skeletal muscles in most species, typically leading to a muscular dystrophy known as white muscle disease. This is exacerbated by high intakes of polyunsaturated fatty acids, and can generally be prevented by increasing the intake of either selenium or vitamin E. In humans selenium deficiency appears mainly to affect the heart, as in the case of a cardiomyopathy known as Keshan disease. This affected a large number of children in the Sichuan province of China until it was found that supplements of sodium selenite would prevent the disease.

Thyroxine 5′-deiodinase catalyses the conversion of the major thyroid hormone thyroxine (T_4) to its more active derivative tri-iodothyronine (T_3) and to the inactive

Selenium is considered as an antioxidant nutrient because of its role in glutathione peroxidase

metabolite reverse T_3. This occurs within the thyroid gland and, more importantly, at the site of action of the hormone in a number of peripheral tissues. It has been studied mainly in the microsomal fraction of the liver. It has been suggested that the ratio of circulating T_3 to T_4 could be a useful index of selenium status, and that selenium status could affect thyroid status in people with marginal iodine intakes.

Selenium enters the body mainly as selenoamino acids, although inorganic selenium can also be absorbed in the small intestine. Meat and fish supply at least 25 per cent of the average intake in this country. Plant sources are rather variable sources of selenium, depending on where the plant was grown. For example, most bread in the UK used to be made from hard wheat imported from North America, which had a high selenium content, but much is now made from home-produced wheat which has a rather lower selenium content.

Selenoamino acids are degraded in the body to inorganic selenium which is excreted in the urine. It is mainly excreted as reduced and methylated derivatives, in amounts which vary in proportion to intake. Thus the selenium status of a population can be determined from plasma or urinary selenium measurements, although it is more reliable to base the assessment of an individual's selenium status on the measurement of glutathione peroxidase activity in tissues such as red blood cells or platelets.

■ 6.4.2 IODINE

The only function of iodine in the body is as a component of the thyroid hormones thyroxine (T_4) and tri-iodothyronine (T_3) (see Figure 6.4). Iodide is taken up into the thyroid gland by an energy-dependent active transport system. Thiocyanate ions can competitively inhibit iodide uptake, and since thiocyanate is generated during the metabolism of hydrogen cyanide, which can be found in cassava, this explains why consumption of cassava can precipitate iodine deficiency when iodine intake is marginal. Iodide enters the colloid between thyroid cells and is oxidized by hydrogen peroxide to iodine. This combines with tyrosine residues in thyroglobulin to form mono- and di-iodotyrosines, and these then couple to form T_3 and T_4. Thioureas irreversibly inhibit the iodination of tyrosine, so that these molecules are also goitrogens, producing similar consequences to thiocyanates. The iodinated thyroglobulin is then taken up into the thyroid cell where proteolytic enzymes release the hormone into the bloodstream. Normally T_4 is secreted in much larger quantities than T_3, but when iodine supply is reduced more T_3 and less T_4 is produced.

Iodine is needed for the synthesis of thyroid hormones

Secretion of thyroid hormones is controlled by thyroid stimulating hormone (TSH) which is released from the pituitary gland. The secretion of TSH in turn is controlled by thyrotropin releasing hormone (TRH) from the hypothalamus, and by feedback from the circulating concentration of T_4. Thus in severe iodine deficiency plasma T_4 levels are low and TSH levels are high. TSH also has a trophic effect on the thyroid gland, and this leads to hypertrophy of the gland when iodine supply is inadequate. An enlarged thyroid gland is known as a goitre, and this is the most characteristic sign of iodine deficiency.

Thyroid hormones stimulate RNA and protein synthesis in a variety of peripheral tissues, with the most noticeable result being an increase in oxygen consumption. They are thus required for the maintenance of adequate rates of energy metabolism, as well as

• **Figure 6.4** Biosynthesis of thyroid hormones

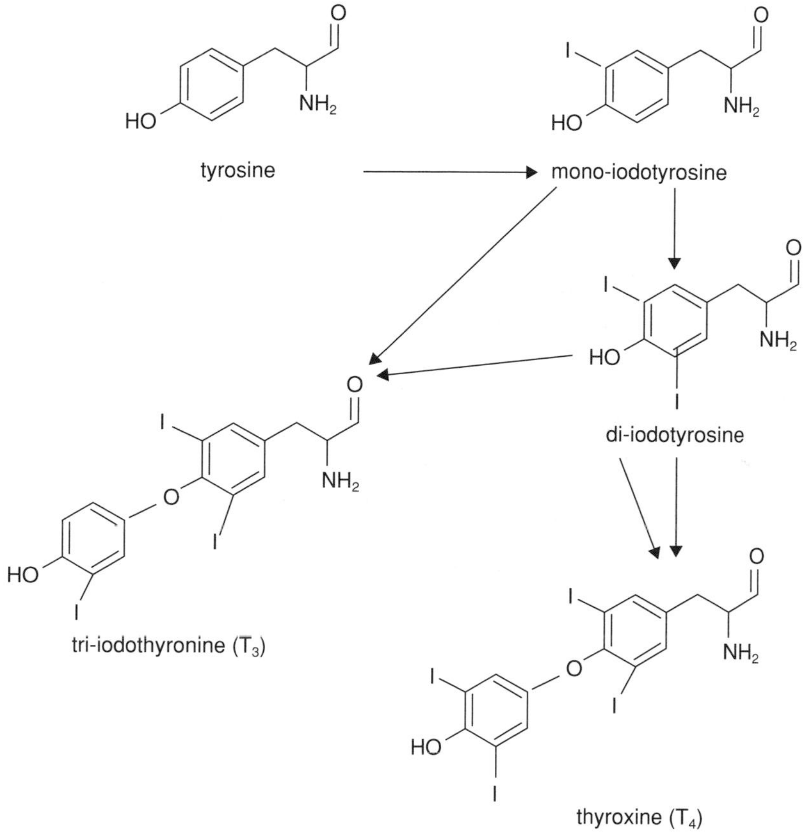

tyrosine → mono-iodotyrosine

di-iodotyrosine

tri-iodothyronine (T₃)

thyroxine (T₄)

normal growth and development. Hence the consequences of hypothyroidism, which may result from iodine deficiency, include lethargy, low work performance and poor cold tolerance. Hypothyroidism will also cause reduced growth rate and developmental retardation, and if this occurs *in utero* it results in cretinism.

The only rich sources of iodine are sea fish, including shellfish, and seaweed. Milk supplies more than one-third of the intake in the UK, although it contains much more iodine in the winter than in the summer because of the seasonal differences in the diets of dairy cattle (cattle feed is supplemented with iodine). The iodine content of plant foods is highly variable, depending on the iodine content of the soil. Thus inland, upland areas which have undergone significant erosion or glaciation are traditionally associated with endemic goitre, particularly if the community is relatively isolated and hence reliant on locally produced food.

Iodide is readily absorbed in the small intestine and efficiently trapped by the thyroid gland, which requires approximately 60 μg/d for hormone synthesis. Thyroid hormones are mainly broken down in the liver, which releases most of the iodide back into the circulation. A small amount is secreted into bile, and thus excreted in the faeces, but most iodine is excreted in urine in amounts that balance intake. Thus the iodide status of a population can be assessed from measurements of urinary iodide excretion or plasma protein-bound iodine concentration, although accurate assessment of individuals requires measurement of specific thyroid hormone levels.

■ 6.4.3 CHROMIUM

Chromium in its trivalent cationic state forms a complex with nicotinic acid and glutathione which is known as the glucose tolerance factor. This appears to facilitate the binding of insulin with its receptor in cell membranes. Thus chromium-deficient patients on long-term total parenteral nutrition show impaired glucose tolerance, high circulating free fatty acid concentrations and weight loss as well as numbness and ataxia, all of which only respond to insulin when chromium supplements are given. However administration of chromium supplements, usually in the form of brewers yeast, to insulin-resistant and diabetic subjects has produced inconsistent results.

Chromium is present in a wide variety of foods, although milling of cereals removes a considerable proportion of it. Less than 1 per cent of inorganic trivalent chromium is absorbed, and although intact glucose tolerance factor is absorbed much more efficiently it also causes an acute increase in urinary chromium excretion. Phytic acid inhibits chromium absorption still further. It is not clear whether absorption improves when chromium status is low. Hexavalent chromium is also absorbed, but is toxic. Plasma chromium concentration does not correlate well with tissue chromium status, and urinary chromium excretion is probably the best indicator of intake, although carbohydrate intake also causes an acute increase in chromium excretion.

Chromium functions as part of the glucose tolerance factor

SUMMARY

- Mineral deficiencies often arise from a failure of absorption or excessive loss.
- Urinary excretion of sodium is tightly controlled to maintain sodium balance over a wide range of intakes.
- Potassium is mainly intracellular, and whole body potassium is a good index of body cell mass.
- Calcium balance is maintained by vitamin D, parathyroid hormone and calcitonin.
- Phosphorus and magnesium deficiencies are rare in humans but more common in farm animals.
- Fluoridation of water at 1 ppm decreases the incidence of dental caries.
- Iron is required for the function of oxygen within the body but too much free iron catalyses the production of damaging free radicals.
- Copper deficiency causes anaemia and, when severe, connective tissue weakness leading to aortic rupture.
- Zinc-dependent enzymes perform hundreds of different functions.
- Selenium is required for the function of glutathione peroxidase, a key antioxidant enzyme.
- Iodine deficiency leading to goitre, hypothyroidism and cretinism is common in inland, upland areas.
- Chromium is part of the glucose tolerance factor which facilitates the binding of insulin to its receptors.

FURTHER READING

British Nutrition Foundation Task Force (1995) *Iron: Nutritional and Physiological Significance*. London: Chapman & Hall.

McCance, R.A. (1936) 'Experimental human salt deficiency', *Lancet*, **i**: 823.

McDowell, L.R. (1992) *Minerals in Animal and Human Nutrition*. New York: Academic Press.

Underwood, E.J. and Mertz, W. (1987) *Trace Elements in Human and Animal Nutrition*. New York: Academic Press.

7

VITAMINS

Vitamins are organic substances which the body requires in small amounts for its metabolism, but which it cannot make for itself in sufficient quantities. A characteristic deficiency disease (such as beri-beri, xerophthalmia or scurvy) develops for many of the vitamins when the supply is inadequate, and this was the original basis for identifying them. Later discoveries were a consequence of understanding the role vitamins play in normal metabolism. Similarly, the assessment of the amounts of each vitamin required were originally based on the amounts required to prevent the deficiency disorder, whereas more recently assessment of requirements has been based on the amount required to permit optimal functioning of particular metabolic pathways. Some vitamins have pharmacological effects when consumed in larger amounts and can be used in the treatment of certain disorders of metabolism. However, some vitamins, particularly vitamins A, D and B_6, are toxic in excess. Consequently, it has become necessary to quantify upper safe limits of intake as well as recommended intakes.

Vitamins can be fat-soluble or water-soluble

There are thirteen vitamins required by humans which can be subdivided into fat-soluble (vitamins A, D, E and K) and water-soluble groups (thiamin (B_1), riboflavin (B_2), niacin, vitamin B_6, biotin, folate, pantothenic acid, vitamins B_{12} and C). There are considerable variations between species in nutrient requirements. There are other compounds which are termed vitamins such as choline, which is required by some other animals but not humans. Similarly, vitamin C (ascorbic acid) is required by humans but not by most other animals. The requirement for vitamins has evolved by the deletion or modification of the genes for the expression of key enzymes. There are some rare human inborn errors of metabolism where replacement of a missing metabolite restores normal functioning, for example in systemic carnitine deficiency. However, carnitine is generally not regarded as an essential vitamin for humans. In the case of vitamin C, where the enzyme L-gulonolactone oxidase is missing, the mutation did not have an impact on the survival of the species when the prehistoric diet contained plenty of fruit and berries, which are a rich source of vitamin C.

The fat-soluble vitamins are found mainly in fatty foods and are less widely distributed than the water-soluble vitamins, and occur in very high concentrations in some foods. For example, cod-liver oil is a rich source of vitamins A and D. With the exception of vitamins B_{12} and C, most water-soluble vitamins are found in a wide variety of foods in moderate amounts. The body can amass stores of vitamins A, D, E and B_{12} which can last months or even years. Yet the capacity for storage for the remaining vitamins is limited and deficiency occurs relatively rapidly on their removal from the diet.

Vitamin deficiencies occur for a variety of reasons: an inadequate dietary intake; malabsorption of the vitamin; increased requirement; and drug-induced deficiency. The classical deficiency diseases such as scurvy, beri-beri, pellagra and xerophthalmia were associated with diets consisting of a limited range of foodstuffs. As dietary diversity increases, the probability of deficiency decreases. In the less economically developed countries where food diversity is limited, the classical nutritional deficiency diseases still occur. In economically developed countries, these classical vitamin deficiency diseases are less common and dietary deficiencies are confined to vagrants, alcoholics and individuals who restrict their diet out of choice or because of loss of appetite. Vitamin deficiency diseases in economically developed countries are more often a consequence of some other disease which leads to malabsorption or increased catabolism or excretion of the vitamin.

> Vitamin deficiencies generally occur when dietary diversity is limited

The nomenclature of the vitamins developed historically as their existence and properties were established. Thus the fat-soluble factor that promoted growth was called vitamin A to distinguish it from the water-soluble factor vitamin B, and this in turn was subdivided into the heat labile vitamin B_1 and the heat stable vitamin B_2, and so on. Where a vitamin has been identified as a single entity, it is now referred to by its chemical name e.g. vitamin B_1 is referred to as thiamin. The alphabetical nomenclature is still useful for those vitamins where a group of related compounds have vitamin activity e.g. vitamin B_6 (pyridoxamine and pyridoxal). It is also useful for describing sources of vitamins in the diet. The term B-complex is often used to describe thiamin, riboflavin, niacin, biotin and vitamin B_6 which occur in similar dietary sources. Some vitamins can be made from other dietary constituents e.g. retinol can be synthesized from β-carotene and niacin from tryptophan. Vitamin D can be synthesized in the skin on exposure to sufficient ultraviolet B light. This does not occur in the winter months from November to February in the UK, so that a dietary intake becomes necessary.

■ 7.1 THIAMIN, NIACIN, RIBOFLAVIN, BIOTIN AND PANTOTHENIC ACID

These B vitamins all function as coenzymes in the central pathways by which fat and carbohydrate are metabolized within the cell. Each is involved in a number of different reactions, so that deficiencies will have a number of different consequences and it is often not clear how these produce particular clinical consequences. They are stored neither by plants nor animals, so there are no particularly rich dietary sources and a regular dietary supply is needed to replace what is lost during normal metabolic turnover. On the other hand, they are present in modest amounts in most foodstuffs. Cereals are the staple foods of most populations and are particularly important sources of these vitamins. The vitamins are concentrated in the aleurone layer of cereal seeds and milling and refining of cereals can lead to large losses. Some of the earliest reports of thiamin deficiency were among prisoners in Java fed on reboiled polished rice. Wholegrain cereals or cereals that have been parboiled before milling retain these vitamins. Yeast is a particularly rich source of these vitamins and where yeast is used in breadmaking, it makes a significant contribution to intake.

B vitamins act mainly as coenzymes

■ 7.1.1 THIAMIN

Thiamin was identified as the vitamin which prevents and cures the deficiency disease beri-beri. The term 'beri-beri' means sheep in Javanese and was used to describe the way in which people afflicted by the disease walked. Classical beri-beri is now rare, but another form of thiamin deficiency called Wernicke-Korsakoff's encephalopathy occurs among alcoholics. For further details on thiamin deficiency see Chapter 8.

7.1.1.1 Functions of thiamin

The main form of thiamin in the body is the diphosphate, which is a coenzyme for oxidative decarboxylation reactions. Three similar multi-enzyme complexes within the mammalian mitochondrion utilize thiamin diphosphate for generating energy. Pyruvate dehydrogenase converts pyruvic acid, which is formed from carbohydrates by glycolysis, into acetyl coenzyme A for entry into the tricarboxylic acid cycle:

$$\text{Pyruvate} + \text{CoASH} + \text{NAD}^+ \rightarrow \text{Acetyl CoA} + \text{CO}_2 + \text{NADH}$$

2-oxoglutarate dehydrogenase is part of the tricarboxylic acid cycle, generating energy from all fuels under aerobic conditions:

$$\text{2-oxoglutarate} + \text{CoASH} + \text{NAD}^+ \rightarrow \text{Succinyl CoA} + \text{CO}_2 + \text{NADH}$$

Branched chain oxo-acid dehydrogenase metabolizes the branched chain amino acids leucine, isoleucine and valine after they have been transaminated. Thus leucine is transaminated to α-oxo-isocaproic acid and this is oxidatively decarboxylated to isovaleryl CoA; isoleucine is transaminated to α-oxo-β-methyl valeric acid and this is oxidatively decarboxylated to α-methylbutyryl CoA; and valine is transaminated to α-oxo-isovaleric acid and this is oxidatively decarboxylated to isobutyryl CoA.

Thiamin diphosphate acts as a coenzyme in oxidative decarboxylation reactions

The binding of thiamin diphosphate to pyruvate dehydrogenase appears to be less tight than its binding to the other two enzymes, and this enzyme is more sensitive to reduced thiamin intake. Thus thiamin deficiency specifically suppresses the aerobic metabolism of carbohydrate, leading to increased production of lactate by glycolysis, and the requirement for thiamin is considered to be greater on a high carbohydrate diet. Because the nervous system has a high demand for ATP generation from carbohydrate the dominant clinical feature of thiamin deficiency is neuropathy. The increase in circulating lactate and pyruvate concentrations after a test dose of glucose has been used to assess thiamin status. Moreover, lactic acidaemia damages the capillaries and dilates the arterioles, leading to the oedema and chronic cardiac failure which are the characteristic features of wet beri-beri.

Thiamin diphosphate is also a cofactor for the transketolase reaction within the pentose phosphate pathway, which is a pathway for the metabolism of glucose to produce NADPH for biosynthetic reactions such as lipogenesis.

ribose-5-phosphate + xylose-5-phosphate

= glyceraldehyde-3-phosphate + sedoheptulose-7-phosphate

The thiamin status of an individual can be assessed by measuring transketolase activity in a sample of their erythrocytes in the presence and absence of additional thiamin diphosphate. If addition of an excess of the cofactor increases enzyme activity by more than 20 per cent the subject is regarded as thiamin deficient. This is an example of a so-called enzyme reactivation test.

A small proportion of the thiamin in the body is present as triphosphate, particularly in the nervous system where it may have a role in conducting impulses by opening chloride channels in the neuronal membrane. Both the central and the peripheral nervous system can be affected by thiamin deficiency, leading to the progressive peripheral neuropathy of dry beri-beri and the confusion and confabulation of the Wernicke-Korsakoff syndrome (see Chapter 8). Several aspects of the functions of thiamin may be involved in these lesions, including the role of thiamin triphosphate in nerve conduction, the role of transketolase in synthesizing myelin lipids, and the role of pyruvate dehydrogenase in generating energy from glucose and in the synthesis of acetyl choline.

Thiamin deficiency mainly affects the nervous system

7.1.1.2 Dietary sources and requirement for thiamin

The requirement for thiamin is closely linked to energy intake, particularly that from carbohydrate. Epidemiological evidence suggests that beri-beri occurs on intakes of less than 0.05 mg/MJ. Depletion and repletion studies show that biochemical indices such as urinary thiamin excretion and the transketolase activation coefficient are normal on intakes of 0.07 mg/MJ, and this is taken as the estimated average requirement. The reference nutrient intake is 0.09 mg/MJ. Mean intakes of adults in the UK are around 0.19 mg/MJ.

Cereal products, especially wholegrain cereals and bread, are the most important sources of thiamin in the UK, accounting for almost 40 per cent of the average intake. In white and brown flour much of the thiamin in wheat is removed during the milling process but in the UK thiamin is added to these flours to restore the level to 0.24 mg/100 g, equivalent to wholemeal flour. Breakfast cereals are also a major source of thiamin because many manufacturers add thiamin (and many other vitamins) to their products voluntarily.

Meat and fish account for 20 per cent of average UK intake, and dairy products another 10 per cent. Potatoes contribute around 17 per cent, with all other vegetables and fruit contributing less than 10 per cent. Thus for thiamin as for most other vitamins, fruit and vegetables are not the major sources. Thiamin is very susceptible to damage at cooking temperatures, particularly in neutral or alkaline solution, and to oxidation by SO_2, which is a common food additive used to kill yeasts.

Thiamin and niacin are added to bread and other wheat products in the UK

■ 7.1.2 NIACIN

Niacin is the term used to describe nicotinic acid and nicotinamide. The vitamin was identified as the heat-stable water-soluble vitamin which prevents and cures the deficiency disease pellagra (which in Spanish means rough skin). Pellagra was a disease that was first observed in Mediterranean countries when the cultivation of maize (a New World crop) as a staple food was introduced. There were epidemic outbreaks in the Deep South of the USA at the beginning of the last century, again associated with overdependence on maize as a staple food. It is still common in parts of Southern Africa and India. Low intakes of niacin have also been linked to an increased risk of nuclear cataract in China and India.

7.1.2.1 Functions of niacin

Niacin functions in the body as the coenzymes NAD (nicotinamide adenine dinucleotide) and NADP (nicotinamide adenine dinucleotide phosphate) in a large number of redox reactions.

NAD is mainly involved in the oxidation of metabolic fuels. The NADH produced is then reoxidized by the mitochondrial electron transport chain. Examples of enzymes which require NAD include pyruvate dehydrogenase, which is involved in the oxidation of carbohydrates, 2-oxoglutarate dehydrogenase and isocitrate dehydrogenase in the citric acid cycle, β-hydroxyacyl dehydrogenase in the β-oxidation pathway of fatty acid oxidation, and alcohol dehydrogenase. Thus NAD is involved in the oxidation of all the major sources of energy in the diet.

In contrast, NADP exists mainly in the reduced form and is involved in biosynthetic pathways such as fatty acid synthesis. It is also used by the enzyme glutathione reductase to maintain glutathione in its reduced form, which is needed as part of the defence against free radicals. Reduced NADP is generated by the pentose phosphate pathway and by the activity of the malic enzyme.

Nicotinamide is metabolized to N^1-methyl nicotinamide and N-methyl pyridone-2-carboxamide. Excretion of these two metabolites in the urine accounts for virtually all the turnover of niacin in the body, and is used as the main biochemical index of niacin status.

Consumption of large amounts (e.g. 100 mg) of nicotinic acid results in flushing of the skin (cutaneous dilatation) and also results in the inhibition of lipolysis by adipose tissue. Nicotinic acid is used as a drug to treat some forms of hyperlipidaemia in doses ranging from 2–3 g/d. The side-effects of skin flush can cause itching but can be relieved by aspirin which suggests that the effects are mediated by prostaglandins or prostacyclin. Nicotinamide is relatively non-toxic in excess but there have been reports of liver failure.

7.1.2.2 Dietary sources and requirement for niacin

Niacin is unique among the water-soluble vitamins in that it can be synthesized within the body. The precursor from which it is synthesized is the essential amino acid tryptophan, and the pathway by which the nicotinamide coenzymes are produced is outlined in Figure 7.1. This is the main pathway of tryptophan metabolism, so that, for an adult in nitrogen balance, the amount of tryptophan available for conversion to nicotinamide coenzymes is equal to about 99 per cent of tryptophan intake. However, under normal conditions NAD and NADP are minor products of the pathway, with most of the tryptophan being converted to acetyl CoA. The proportion of tryptophan actually converted to nicotinamide coenzymes varies quite widely, and it is conventional to assume that 60 mg tryptophan is equivalent to 1 mg of preformed niacin when evaluating dietary sources of niacin. The amount of niacin potentially available from food calculated in this way is known as 'niacin equivalents'.

NAD and NADP are redox carriers derived from niacin

Niacin can be synthesized from tryptophan in the body

• **Figure 7.1** Conversion of tryptophan to NAD and NADP

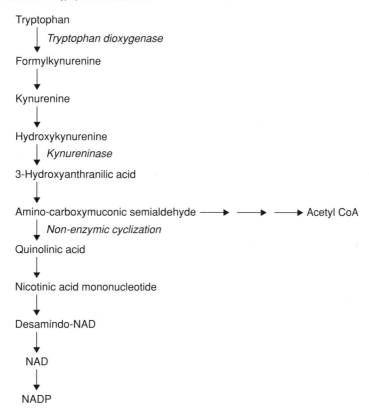

About half the niacin equivalents in the UK diet come from preformed nicotinic acid and nicotinamide. About 40 per cent of this comes from meat, and another 20 per cent from vegetables. Cereal grains also contain significant amounts of preformed niacin, but much of this is believed to be bound in a form which is biologically unavailable. On the other hand, the leavening process during bread making probably releases some of this niacin, and synthetic niacin is added by law to all wheat flour (except wholemeal) and voluntarily to most breakfast cereals. The other half of the niacin equivalents come from the tryptophan in the major sources of protein, i.e. meat, dairy products and cereals. Total intakes of niacin equivalents are around 35 mg/d for adults in this country, or approximately 200 per cent of the reference nutrient intake.

■ 7.1.3 RIBOFLAVIN

Riboflavin was initially identified as the heat stable vitamin B_2. Deficiency of riboflavin does not appear to cause any fatal disease, but large numbers of people around the world are probably at least marginally deficient in the vitamin. The consequences of deficiency are skin lesions particularly of mucous membranes of the reproductive organs and at the angles of the mouth (angular stomatitis). Low intakes have also been linked to an increased incidence of nuclear cataracts (a cause of blindness).

Riboflavin deficiency is widespread but is generally not fatal

7.1.3.1 Functions of riboflavin

Riboflavin functions in the body as two similar coenzymes, riboflavin 5′-phosphate (commonly known as flavin mononucleotide, FMN) and flavin adenine dinucleotide, FAD. Like the nicotinamide coenzymes these are involved in a large number of redox reactions, including the production of energy from all the major fuels. However they are much more tightly bound to their apoenzymes than other vitamin-derived coenzymes, in some cases being covalently bound, so that these enzymes are known as flavoproteins.

Flavoproteins are redox enzymes derived from riboflavin

Riboflavin phosphate provides the link between substrate level oxidation and the mitochondrial electron transport chain. NAD is reduced by pyruvate dehydrogenase or by 2-oxoglutarate dehydrogenase or isocitrate dehydrogenase in the citric acid cycle. The electrons are passed on to riboflavin phosphate, with the generation of ATP, and thence to ubiquinone and the electron transport chain, where two more molecules of ATP are generated and oxygen is reduced to water.

Most other enzymes use FAD. These include succinate dehydrogenase in the citric acid cycle, which passes electrons on directly to ubiquinone and thus generates only two molecules of ATP, and fatty acyl CoA dehydrogenase, the first step in the β-oxidation of fatty acids. There are also several enzymes which oxidize molecular oxygen directly, including xanthine oxidase, retinal oxidase and amino acid oxidases.

Another important flavoprotein is glutathione reductase, which maintains glutathione in its reduced form to protect the cell against oxidative damage. The activity of this enzyme can be measured in vitro in red blood cells, and this forms the basis of another enzyme reactivation test, the erythrocyte glutathione reductase activation coefficient (EGRAC) test for riboflavin status. If addition of excess FAD increases the activity of the enzyme by more than 30 per cent the subject is judged to be riboflavin deficient. Riboflavin status can also be assessed from the urinary excretion of riboflavin.

7.1.3.2 Dietary sources and requirement for riboflavin

Riboflavin is much less widely distributed than most of the other B vitamins. In particular cereals contribute only 22 per cent of the average intake in the UK, and half of this is from fortified breakfast cereals; bread is not routinely fortified with riboflavin in the UK although it is in some other countries. Milk is the most important source, supplying on average 27 per cent, with meat supplying 21 per cent while fruit and vegetables account for only 8 per cent. The diets of many poor communities in developing countries contain very little milk or meat, so their riboflavin contents are likely to be rather low.

Milk is the major source of riboflavin in the UK

Riboflavin is relatively stable when heated and thus during most cooking and food processing, but it is sensitive to visible light. Although only the surface layers of a product may be affected by this it could be important where riboflavin intakes are marginal.

Average intakes of riboflavin in the UK are 2.1 mg/d for adult men and 1.6 mg/d for adult women, only 40 per cent above the RNI and thus more marginal than most other B vitamins. Moreover, there is a considerable social class gradient, with intakes in classes 1 and 2 being 35 per cent greater than those in classes 4 and 5. A survey of apparently healthy British adults found biochemical evidence of marginal riboflavin deficiency (an EGRAC value greater than 1.3) in 1 per cent of men and 2 per cent of women.

■ 7.1.4 BIOTIN

Biotin is an essential growth factor for many organisms but it is so widely distributed in foods that deficiency in humans is extremely rare. However, refined cereal products, fruit and root crops are relatively poor sources. There may also be some absorption of biotin synthesized by bacteria in the lower gut. Thus the only reported cases of deficiency arising from inadequate intake in humans have occurred in patients maintained on long-term total parenteral nutrition following major bowel resection. Deficiency symptoms include a dry scaly skin, dermatitis, loss of appetite, vomiting, muscle pains and inflammation of the tongue (glossitis). Isolated deficiencies have also occurred in individuals consuming bizarre diets containing large amounts of raw eggs (12 or more per day). This is because raw egg white contains a glycoprotein called avidin which binds to biotin and renders it unavailable for absorption. Cooking the eggs denatures the avidin and renders it harmless.

Avidin binds to biotin and prevents its absorption from the gut

Biotin functions as a coenzyme in carboxylation reactions by acting as a carrier for carbon dioxide. Thus biotin-dependent enzymes include pyruvate carboxylase, which initiates the pathway of gluconeogenesis, and acetyl CoA carboxylase which produces malonyl CoA to initiate fatty acid synthesis. A similar reaction is the conversion of propionic acid to methylmalonyl CoA, which is particularly important in the synthesis of glucose in ruminant animals (cows, goats and sheep). Biotin deficiency in poultry results in sudden death on exposure to stress; a result of low blood glucose concentration (hypoglycaemia) and accumulation of fat in the liver and kidney. It was suggested that a marginal biotin intake may be linked to cot-death in infants but this has never been substantiated.

■ 7.1.5 PANTOTHENIC ACID

As its name suggests, pantothenic acid is also extremely widely distributed in foods. No cases of pure pantothenic acid deficiency have ever been confirmed in free living subjects. Deficiency symptoms ("burning feet syndrome") have been produced in volunteers fed semi-synthetic diets depleted of pantothenic acid or to which an antagonist to pantothenic acid has been added.

Pantothenic acid is the main component of coenzyme A. It is thus involved in many pathways of intermediary metabolism, including both the synthesis and the breakdown of fatty acids and the oxidation of carbohydrates.

■ 7.2 VITAMIN B$_{12}$, FOLATE AND VITAMIN B$_6$

These vitamins play an important role as coenzymes in the 1-carbon cycle and in the metabolism of amino and nucleic acids. They have in common some of the metabolic consequences of deficiency e.g. elevations in plasma homocysteine concentration (see Figure 7.2).

■ 7.2.1 VITAMIN B$_6$

Vitamin B$_6$ exists in three major chemical forms: pyridoxine, pyridoxal, and pyridoxamine. These are all precursors to pyridoxal phosphate, a coenzyme for several important reactions involved in protein metabolism, including the transamination reactions necessary for synthesis of amino acids. Dietary deficiency of vitamin B$_6$ is rare and signs of deficiency include dermatitis, glossitis, anaemia, depression, confusion, and convulsions. Good dietary sources of the vitamin include fish, lean meat, wholegrain cereals, bananas, beans and peanut butter.

Pyridoxal phosphate, derived from vitamin B$_6$, is a cofactor for transamination reactions

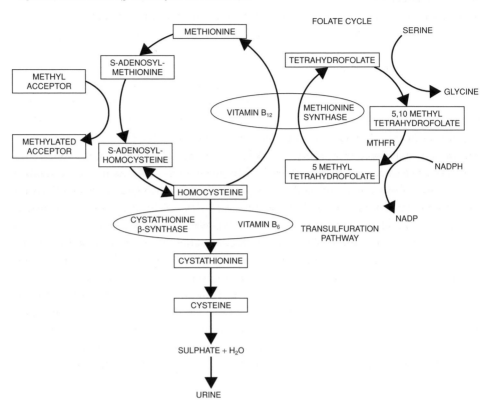

• **Figure 7.2** Folate, vitamin B_{12}, vitamin B_6 and the 1-carbon cycle

7.2.1.1 Metabolic role of vitamin B_6

Pyridoxal phosphate is a coenzyme for transamination and deamination reactions. It is also involved in the decarboxylation reaction necessary for the synthesis of serotonin, noradrenaline and histamine from tryptophan, tyrosine and histidine respectively. It is required as a cofactor in the kynureninase reaction involved in the synthesis of niacin from tryptophan and is also a cofactor in the transulphuration pathway where it can transfer the sulphydryl group from methionine to serine or from homocysteine to cystathionine. Pyridoxine can modify the action of steroid hormones *in vivo* by interacting with steroid-receptor complexes. Pyridoxine is also essential for the manufacture of prostaglandins and haemoglobin.

Although pyridoxine deficiency is rare, pyridoxine is an approved treatment for sideroblastic anaemias, where the incorporation of iron into the haem molecule is impaired, and pyridoxine-dependent inborn errors of the metabolism such as cystathionine β-synthase deficiency. Pyridoxine has also been claimed to alleviate the symptoms of premenstrual syndrome, pregnancy sickness, carpal tunnel syndrome, hyperhomocystinaemia (a risk factor for cardiovascular disease) and neuropathies. However, excessive intake of the vitamin (more than 50 mg/d) have been shown to result in sensory peripheral neuropathy which is generally reversible following cessation of taking the supplement. Very high intakes in the order of 2–3 g/d may result in permanent nerve damage.

Recommended intakes of pyridoxine are based on protein intake. In the UK, the RNI is set at 15 µg/g protein for adults. This is equivalent to approximately 1.4 and 1.2 mg/d in the UK for males and females respectively.

■ 7.2.2 VITAMIN B₁₂

Vitamin B_{12} is needed for normal blood formation and neurological functioning. Deficiency most commonly results from an inability to absorb the vitamin properly rather than a lack of the vitamin in the diet and may affect between 5–15 per cent of the elderly population in the UK. Vitamin B_{12} is unique among the vitamins in that its primary source is of microbiological origin. Plant foods are free from the vitamin unless contaminated with bacteria that produce it. The main source of vitamin B_{12} in human diets is animal products, although small amounts may be obtained from microbiologically contaminated water in developing countries. Vitamin B_{12} in animal tissues is derived from the consumption of microbes (especially in fish and shellfish), from microbial flora in the intestinal tract in ruminants (sheep, cows and goats) or from coprophagy (eating faeces) e.g. in rabbits. Fish, particularly shellfish, are the richest food sources but quantitatively meat is more important because it is consumed in larger amounts. Vitamin B_{12} is stored in the liver and kidney and so is found in high concentrations in these foods. It is also found in lower amounts in milk, cheese and eggs. Food tables suggest that some fermented foods such as tempeh (fermented soybeans) and beer contain the vitamin but this may be in a form that is not biologically active. Some fermentation processes destroy the vitamin, for example yoghurt is free from vitamin B_{12}.

Vitamin B_{12} is present only in foods of animal or microbial origin

7.2.2.1 Metabolic role of vitamin B₁₂

The term vitamin B_{12} refers to all members of a group of large cobalt-containing corinoids that can be converted into methyl cobalamin and adenosyl cobalamin, the two main cobalamin-containing coenzymes. The coenzyme methyl cobalamin is a cofactor for methionine synthase which methylates homocysteine to methionine, with methyl-tetrahydrofolate as the methyl group donor (Figure 7.2). This action releases the unmethylated folate cofactor for other single carbon transfer reactions important in nucleic acid synthesis. In vitamin B_{12} deficiency the concentration of homocysteine (Hcy) in plasma is increased. One of the major consequences of a deficiency of vitamin B_{12} is a reduction in the availability of folate for its essential role in DNA synthesis. This is called the 'methyl folate trap' and results in impaired cell division. It can, however, be overcome if the intake of folate is increased. Hence the consequences of vitamin B_{12} deficiency are strongly dependent on the intake of folate.

The other major cobalamin coenzyme, adenosylcobalamin, catalyses mutase reactions in which a hydrogen and some group on an adjacent carbon exchange places (these include glutamate mutase, ornithine mutase, L-β-lysine mutase, leucine amino mutase and methyl malonyl mutase). The conversion of methyl malonyl coenzyme A to succinyl coenzyme A is an important step in the pathway for the degradation of certain amino acids and odd chain fatty acids. In deficiency, the concentration of methyl malonic acid (MMA) in plasma is increased. Thus elevations of plasma MMA and Hcy concentrations can be used as indices of vitamin B_{12} status.

7.2.2.2 Causes and consequences of vitamin B_{12} deficiency

Dietary vitamin B_{12} deficiency often occurs in vegans and vegetarians but generally not in a severe form. In meat eaters deficiency most commonly results from an inability to absorb the vitamin and is termed pernicious anaemia. This is usually a consequence of antibodies to, or an impaired ability to produce, the intrinsic factor which is needed for the absorption of the vitamin. Intrinsic factor is secreted by parietal cells in the stomach, and absorption of the vitamin B_{12}–intrinsic factor complex occurs in the last 30 cm of the ileum. Consequently, surgical removal of the stomach or the terminal ileum will result in a failure to absorb the vitamin. Deficiency can also be caused by the intestinal parasite *Diphyllobothrium latum* (the fish tape worm).

Vitamin B_{12} deficiency results in macrocytic megaloblastic anaemia, neurological symptoms due to demyelination of the spinal cord, brain and optic and peripheral nerves and other less specific symptoms, such as sore tongue and weakness. Pernicious anaemia requires treatment by intramuscular injections of vitamin B_{12}. If patients with pernicious anaemia are given high intakes of folic acid, it corrects the anaemia but allows the more insidious neurological complications to progress which can lead to paralysis and death. This is termed the 'masking' of vitamin B_{12} deficiency by folate. Dietary vitamin B_{12} deficiency can also occur in breastfed infants, secondary to a maternal deficiency.

Vitamin B_{12} status can be assessed by measuring the concentration in plasma (which should be in excess of 200 ng/L) and by undertaking full blood counts. Plasma Hcy and MMA concentrations can be used as more sensitive markers of vitamin B_{12} status. The requirement for vitamin B_{12} is very small, about 0.5–1.0 μg/d and the UK RNI is 1.5 μg/d. Average intakes in the UK among omnivores are about 4–6 μg. Fairly regular intake – at least 3 times a week – is desirable as it is not possible to absorb more than 3 μg of any dose taken by mouth.

Vitamin B_{12} deficiency causes megaloblastic anaemia and more serious neurological damage

■ 7.2.3 FOLATE

The term folacin is used to describe a family of compounds called the folates. In the body, the main naturally occurring forms are tetrahydrofolate (THF), 5-methyl THF and 10-formyltetrahydrofolate. Polyglutamate forms of 5-MeTHF predominate in fresh food. These can be broken down by gamma-glutamyl hydrolase in the intestine. The main circulating form is monoglutamate 5-MeTHF which is stored in the liver. The synthetic form of the vitamin is called folic acid and is converted to THF following absorption. Naturally occuring dietary sources of folate have polyglutamate side chains of varying length and require the action of a conjugase enzyme in the intestine to release the active form of the vitamin. Yeast and yeast extracts, e.g. Marmite™ are the richest sources of folate, and significant amounts are supplied by dark green vegetables. Wholegrain cereals are also important sources of the vitamin. However, fortified breakfast cereals and margarine have now become important sources of folic acid in the diet.

7.2.3.1 Metabolic role of folate

Within cells, folate is retained in the cytoplasm by polyglutamation. 5-Methyl-THF is not a good substrate for polyglutamation, and must be first converted, via a vitamin B_{12}-dependent reaction, to THF. Alternatively, folic acid can be converted to polyglutamate (i.e. metabolically active) forms via a vitamin B_{12}-independent pathway. 5-MeTHF is a cofactor for the remethylation of methionine and if the supply is inadequate the concentration of homocysteine increases. If the methylation cycle is impaired, this can result in decreased methylation of DNA which may affect gene transcription. THF is required for the synthesis of deoxyuridine, a component of nucleic acids. Folate deficiency results in reduced *de novo* DNA biosynthesis and, thus, impairment of cell replication, with the most obvious effects relating to rapidly dividing cell types such as erythrocytes and other cells generated by the bone marrow, enterocytes and skin cells. Hence folate deficiency causes a megaloblastic and macrocytic anaemia. Other rapidly regenerating tissues may suffer such as the intestinal villi and the tongue which appears smooth and sore. Experimental deficiency is also accompanied by forgetfulness and irritability.

Folate deficiency causes megaloblastic anaemia

Folate status can be assessed by measuring the level in the serum or better still in erythrocytes which tend to reflect hepatic stores. Experimental folate deficiency can be cured by as little as 50 μg/d and doses in the range of 50–100 μg/d cure naturally occurring megaloblastic anaemia. In developed countries, 8–10 per cent of the population have low concentrations of erythrocyte folate implying that they have low stores. In the UK, median intakes in men are 300 μg/d and in women 200 μg/d. The RNI is 200 μg/d for both men and women. There is an increased requirement for folate during pregnancy owing to increased cell synthesis associated with the growth of the placenta and foetus and megaloblastic anaemia is more likely to occur in late pregnancy.

An additional intake of at least 200 μg/d folic acid in early pregnancy has been found to prevent neural tube defects such as spina bifida. However, to be effective the additional folic acid must be consumed within the first two months of pregnancy. The Department of Health currently advises all women who may become pregnant to consume an additional 400 μg/d folic acid to prevent neural tube defects. For those who have already given birth to one child with a NTD the recommendation is to consume 4–5 mg/d folic acid in the periconceptional period.

Folic acid supplements are recommended before and during early pregnancy to help prevent neural tube defects

Folate deficiency can also occur due to disease of the small bowel, for example in tropical sprue or other enteropathy. Folate deficiency can result from treatment with the drug methotrexate, which is a specific folate antagonist. The drug is used to treat psoriasis and is widely used in cancer chemotherapy because it decreases cell synthesis.

Folate is subject to quite large losses during cooking, especially as it is water soluble. The elderly may be at risk from folate deficiency because of a restricted dietary intake and institutionalized food. Many breakfast cereals and some breads are voluntarily fortified with folic acid. In the USA, all flour is now mandatorily fortified with folic acid at a level of 140 μg/100 g. Fortification is voluntary in the UK as there is concern that compulsory fortification may result in the masking of pernicious anaemia leading to the more insidious neurological signs. Others argue that an increased intake of folic acid could decrease the risk of cardiovascular disease by decreasing plasma Hcy concentration.

■ 7.3 VITAMIN C

Vitamin C is only required by a few species which are referred to as the dependent species and which include humans, primates, the fruit bat, the guinea pig, the red-vented bulbul or turkey and certain salmon. Active forms of the vitamin are L-ascorbic acid and L-dehydroascorbic acid. The dependent species lack L-gulonolactone oxidase and cannot synthesize ascorbic acid from glucose.

Vitamin C is absent from cereal foods and only found in very low concentrations in milk and meat. The most important dietary sources are potatoes, citrus fruit and leafy vegetables such as cabbage. Because it is an antioxidant, vitamin C is very susceptible to oxidation by either enzymic or non-enzymic mechanisms, so a considerable proportion of its activity can be lost during storage, food preparation or processing, particularly where heating is involved. It is also susceptible to loss by leaching into the cooking or processing water.

Vitamin C is very susceptible to loss during food processing

Deficiency results in scurvy which is characterized by impaired wound healing, perifollicular haemorrhages (petechiae), mental confusion, lassitude and fatigue. Scurvy was first accurately described among sailors in medieval times, when ships' rations were devoid of fresh fruit and vegetables, and potatoes, which originate from the New World, had yet to become a staple food. Indeed, the voyages of discovery were limited by the vitamin C content of the rations and scurvy was the major cause of death. Scurvy can be prevented by as little as 10 mg vitamin C/d and as average intakes are now in excess of 60 mg/d it is not surprising that it is nowadays rare. The RNI for the vitamin is 40 mg/d in adults and this is based on the amount needed to maintain plasma concentrations above 0.2 mg/dl. However, occasional cases have been reported in elderly people living on a diet of tea and biscuits. Of more concern is the issue of suboptimal intakes that may influence resistance to infection and wound healing. Several large studies have investigated the effects of vitamin C supplementation on the health of the elderly, and demonstrate neither benefit nor harm.

■ 7.3.1 METABOLIC ROLE OF VITAMIN C

Vitamin C is a water-soluble anti-oxidant and facilates several hydroxylation reactions. In deficiency, the hydroxylation of proline is impaired and this results in defects in the tertiary structure of collagen, which makes up the intercellular matrix and wound tissue. This partially explains the poor wound healing in scurvy. There is also impaired conversion of 3,4-dihydroxyphenylethylamine to noradrenaline. Noradrenaline is an important neurotransmitter in the central nervous system but also plays an important role in maintaining vascular tone. The failure to produce adequate amounts of noradrenaline may also help explain the bleeding tendency as well as some of the pyschiatric symptoms of scurvy.

■ 7.4 FAT-SOLUBLE VITAMINS A, D, E AND K

As their name implies, these compounds are soluble in lipids and are often found in foods high in fat and require the presence of fat for their absorption. If the absorption of fat is impaired then so is the absorption of these vitamins. As they are fat-soluble they are not as easily excreted from the body. With the exception of vitamin K, there are significant body stores of the vitamins and so it is less important to ensure frequent intake than for water-soluble vitamins. Both vitamins A and D have direct effects on gene transcription and are very toxic when consumed in excess.

■ 7.4.1 VITAMIN A

Vitamin A is required for normal vision, growth and cellular differentiation. Deficiency of vitamin A is a major cause of blindness in developing countries and also contributes to impaired immune function resulting in increased mortality from childhood diseases such

• **Figure 7.3** Metabolism of vitamin A

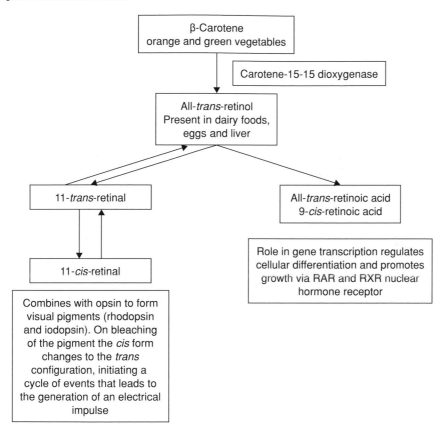

as measles. Vitamin A is the term used to describe all-*trans*-retinol, which is found in animal products such as egg yolk, dairy fat and liver, and its precursors (carotenoid pigments) which are found in orange, red and green vegetables. The retinol molecule consists of a β-ionone ring with an isoprenylated side chain containing a series of conjugated double bonds, which function to absorb energy from photons. The major carotenoid pigment in the diet is β-carotene, which is effectively two retinol molecules joined together. Retinol has an alcohol group at the end of the side chain which undergoes oxidative metabolism to form 11-*cis*-retinal, all-*trans*-retinoic acid and 9-*cis*-retinoic acid (Figure 7.3).

Dietary sources of retinol are usually present in fat-containing foods e.g. liver, egg yolk and butter, and are well absorbed. In contrast carotenoids are generally present in low fat foods (e.g. carrots and dark green vegetables) and are poorly absorbed (on average only 30 per cent is absorbed). However, the absorption of carotenoids is increased if the vegetables are puréed or cooked in fat. Some carotene is converted to retinol in the intestinal wall by a 15,15-dioxygenase but the efficiency of conversion is such that one mole of β-carotene results in one mole of retinol. Consequently only 1/6 of the carotene in the diet is converted to retinol. A system of retinol equivalents is used to estimate total vitamin A intake which allows for the lower bioavailability of carotenoids. In its simplest form it is as follows:

Vitamin A is obtained from animal products as retinol or by conversion of carotenes from plant foods

$$\text{Dietary intake in retinol equivalents (r.e.)} = \mu\text{g retinol in diet} + \frac{\mu\text{g }\beta\text{-carotene in diet}}{6}$$

Dietary reference values for vitamin A are expressed in retinol equivalent. The RNI is 700 r.e./d for adult males, 600 r.e./d for adult women and 350 r.e./d for infants. As vitamin A is stored in the liver, a daily intake is not required. However, intake exceeding 3,300 r.e./d should be avoided by women of reproductive age as an excessive intake has been linked to an increased risk of birth defects such as cleft palate. Vitamin A deficiency disease (VADD) is a major public health problem affecting children in the age range of 1–6 years in developing countries. It is relatively uncommon in adults as beyond the age of 6 years most individuals have significant stores of the vitamin in their liver that can tide them over during periods of food shortage.

Retinol itself plays no specific physiological role but its metabolites do: **retinal** is involved in the visual process and **retinoic acid** is important for regulating gene expression which results in cellular differentiation. It has recently been suggested that carotenoid pigments, besides being precursors for retinol, may have a specific role in protecting against oxidative damage in tissues, especially the eye.

7.4.1.1 Role of vitamin A in the visual process

Mild vitamin A deficiency affects dark adaptation and leads to an increased risk of death from measles but more severe deficiency causes blindness

The photoreceptor cells in the eye are located in the retina and can be divided into two classes: rods (which are responsible for detecting vision in low light intensity and movement); and cones (which are responsible for high acuity and colour vision). Both types of cells contain pigments which themselves contain derivatives of vitamin A. The light responsive pigment in the rods is termed rhodopsin (visual purple) and those in cones are called iodopsins (with sensitivities for red, green and blue wavelengths); these are a complex between 11-*cis*-retinal and opsin. 11-*cis*-retinal is formed in the retina from 11-*cis*-retinol which in turn is derived from all-*trans*-retinol. The *cis*-configuration allows the retinal to fit into a cleft in the opsin protein and the purple colour can be ascribed to the resonance of the conjugated double bond system of 11-*cis*-retinal. When a photon interacts with rhodopsin, the configuration of 11-*cis*-retinal changes to 11-*trans*-retinal. The *cis-trans* isomerization causes the retinal to dissociate from opsin (bleaching of the pigment) and results in the release of energy and membrane depolarization which is transmitted via bipolar cells to the optic nerve. The activated rhodopsin repeatedly contacts molecules of the heterotrimeric G protein, catalysing the exchange of GDP with GTP, producing the active form Gα-GTP. Two of the Gα-GTP sub-units bind to two inhibitory sub-units of phosphodiesterase which then catalyses the hydrolysis of cGMP. The consequent reduction in the cytoplasmic concentration of cGMP leads to the closure of the cyclic-nucleotide gated channels and blockage of the inwards flux of Na^+ and Ca^{2+} (thereby reducing the circulating electrical current). 11-*cis*-retinal is regenerated within the retina but is strongly dependent upon a continued supply from the plasma. This is why night blindness (nyctalopia) is one of the earliest signs of vitamin A deficiency disease.

7.4.1.2 Role of vitamin A in regulating growth and cellular differentiation

Retinol is oxidized irreversibly to all-*trans*-retinoic acid. This metabolite is responsible for the growth promoting effects of vitamin A and acts directly upon the expression of

• **Figure 7.4** Role of vitamin A in gene transcription

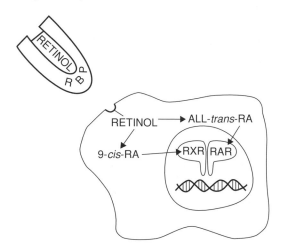

DNA via specific nuclear receptors – the RXR and RAR receptors (Figure 7.4). All-*trans*-retinoic acid is the ligand for the RAR receptor and 9-*cis*-retinoic acid is the main ligand for the RXR receptor. The RXR:RAR heterodimer binds to a retinoic acid response element which results in a motif that causes gene transcription. The RXR receptor acts as a partner for the vitamin D, PPAR and LXR receptors. Retinoic acid plays an important role in embryogenesis by interacting with homeotic (HOX) genes and both a lack of retinoic acid as well as an excess results in abnormal cellular differentiation. Each HOX cluster has a response element to retinoic acid. This is why both a deficiency of vitamin A and an excess results in birth (teratogenic) defects.

The levels of vitamin A in tissues are regulated very carefully by binding proteins, and excess vitamin A is stored in the liver in stellate cells as retinyl esters by the action of lecithin retinol acyl transferase (LRAT). This enzyme esterifies the fatty acid on the *sn*-1 position of lecithin, which is usually palmitic acid, onto retinol: this is why liver contains mainly retinyl palmitate. Retinyl esters are very non-polar and so are stored in fat droplets within the cell. This is an important mechanism for regulating the amount of free retinol in the cell. Retinol can be released by the action of retinyl ester hydrolase. Retinol is transported to tissues bound to retinol binding protein (RBP). This prevents the retinol being oxidized in the circulation to its active metabolite retinoic acid. RBP delivers retinol to cells where it is taken up by specific receptors, and intracellularly retinol and retinoic acid are transported by specific binding proteins which deliver retinoic acid to the nuclear hormone receptors that regulate gene transcription. Deficiency of vitamin A is charac-terized by widespread impairment of growth and cellular differentiation and this is first observed in tissues with high rates of cell turnover such as epithelial tissues, particularly the mucous membranes in the eye, and the respiratory and digestive tracts. One particular feature is a failure of epithelial cells to differentiate and form goblet cells which produce mucus. Instead, columnar epithelial cells stack up on top of each other, resulting in the drying up of mucous membranes and the formation of plaques of keratin (the main protein in skin).

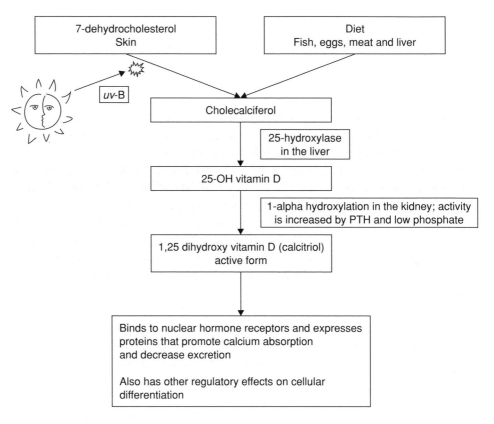

• **Figure 7.5** Metabolism of vitamin D

■ 7.4.2 VITAMIN D

Vitamin D is not required in the diet if exposure to sunlight is adequate. Vitamin D is the precursor of steroid hormones involved in regulating calcium and phosphate homeostasis and is synthesized in the skin following exposure to uv-B radiation. In this reaction cholecalciferol is synthesized from 7-dehydrocholesterol. Cholecalciferol has no vitamin activity until it undergoes 25-hydroxylation in the liver to form 25-OH cholecalciferol and then activation to 1, 25-dihydroxycholecalciferol, which is the fully active form of the vitamin (Figure 7.5). Plasma 1, 25 (OH) vitamin D concentrations are determined by 1-alpha hydroxylase activity in the kidney. This is the main site of 1-alpha hydroxylase, but many cells possess the enzyme. Hepatic synthesis of 25-hydroxycholecalciferol is only loosely regulated, and blood levels reflect the amount of vitamin D endogenously synthesized or obtained from the diet. The half-life of 25-(OH) cholecalciferol in blood is several weeks, whereas that of 1, 25-(OH)$_2$ cholecalciferol is only a few hours. The activity of 1-alpha-hydroxylase in the kidney is tightly regulated and serves as the major control point in production of the active hormone. The major inducer of 1-alpha-hydroxylase is parathyroid hormone (PTH) but it can also be induced by low blood levels of phosphate.

The active form of vitamin D is regarded as a hormone

Vitamin D stimulates the expression of calbindin, an intracellular protein that ferries calcium across the intestinal epithelial cells. In common with other steroid hormones, the vitamin D receptor binds to intracellular receptors that then function as transcription factors to modulate gene expression. The vitamin D receptor has hormone-binding and DNA-binding domains. It forms a complex with another intracellular receptor, the RXR receptor, and that heterodimer is what binds to DNA. The affinity of the vitamin D receptor for 1, 25-(OH)$_2$-cholecalciferol is roughly 1,000 times that for 25-OH-cholecalciferol. Besides stimulating calcium binding proteins, 1, 25-(OH)$_2$-cholecalciferol also acts as a transcriptional regulator of bone matrix proteins; it induces the expression of osteocalcin and suppresses the synthesis of type I collagen. It also induces differentiation of osteoclasts, which are critical for bone remodelling. A variety of cells have been shown to possess 1-alpha hydroxylase activity, e.g. endothelial cells, prostate cells, skin, macrophages and bone. It is believed that locally synthesized 1, 25-(OH)$_2$-cholecalciferol has paracrine functions within these tissues. However, its main physiological role is to provide bone with a proper balance of calcium and phosphorus for bone mineralization.

Adequate amounts of cholecalciferol are synthesized by exposure of the cheeks of the face to 10 minutes of strong sunlight each day. However, a sunscreen of greater than SPF 8 prevents vitamin D synthesis. Cholecalciferol synthesized during the summer months can be stored in the liver and adipose tissue to tide over the winter months. In the UK there is very little synthesis of vitamin D in the months of November to February. There are two dietary forms of vitamin D: cholecalciferol, which is found in meat and particularly oily fish, and ergocalciferol, a fungal steroid which has vitamin activity and is used in vegetarian foods. An intake of up to 10 μg/d is recommended in children and in adults where there is no exposure to sunlight. Margarine and yellow fat spreads are fortified with 79.4 μg/kg in the UK by law and some breakfast cereals are also fortified with the vitamin on a voluntary basis.

Deficiency of vitamin D results in rickets (characterized by bow legs and knock knees) in children and osteomalacia (painful bones) in adults (see Chapter 8). Rickets is now fortunately uncommon but there have been outbreaks among the Asian population and some vegan families in the UK. Rickets currently affects a high proportion of children in Middle-Eastern countries and in urban China. The cause of rickets in these countries is complex and is not simply a consequence of low exposure to sunlight but also low availability of calcium from the diet caused by phytic acid (see Chapter 6).

Rickets most commonly occurs among children during the first five years of life, although it can also occur during adolescence. Premature infants are particularly prone to rickets, and maternal vitamin D deficiency can cause fetal rickets. Biochemical markers of rickets include low plasma 25-OH-cholecalciferol concentrations, increased parathyroid hormone, a mild elevation of alkaline phosphatase and an increase in the bone isoenzyme of 5-nucleotidase. Diagnosis needs to be confirmed by X-ray. Values of 25-OH vitamin cholecalciferol below 4 ng/ml (10 nmol/l) are regarded as deficient, although such levels may not always be accompanied by clinical rickets. Rickets can also occur due to a deficiency of 1-alpha-hydroxylase activity either because of kidney disease or an inborn error of metabolism. This form responds to 1-OH cholecalciferol. It has been argued that higher plasma concentrations of 25-OH vitamin D of around 80 nmol/l are desirable as they are associated with a lower risk of some cancers, especially prostate cancer. However, sunlight exposure is the major determinant of plasma 25-OH vitamin cholecalciferol concentrations rather than diet.

Vitamin D deficiency causes rickets in children and osteomalacia in adults

Excessive intakes of vitamin D (usually above 250 µg/d) can cause hypercalcaemia (toxicity caused by high blood levels of calcium) as a result of increased absorption of calcium. This can result in the deposition of calcium in soft tissues including the heart, lung and tubules of the kidney and may ultimately prove fatal.

■ 7.4.3 VITAMIN K

Vitamin K consists of a group of quinone compounds called phylloquinones, which are found in plants, and menaquinones, which are of bacterial origin. It appears that a significant proportion of vitamin K intake may be derived from bacterial intestinal synthesis. Dietary sources of the vitamin are ubiquitous and some vegetable oils such as corn oil are rich sources. A synthetic form of the vitamin menadione, which lacks the side chain, has complete vitamin activity. Deficiency of vitamin K is characterized by a bleeding disorder which can result in internal haemorrhaging. Dietary deficiency is virtually unknown but can occur in patients undergoing parenteral nutrition. In these patients an intake of 1 µg/kg body weight appears to prevent deficiency. Vitamin K is routinely administered to children at birth, usually 1 mg intramuscularly to prevent haemorrhagic disease of the newborn. Intakes in adults are around 300–500 µg/d compared with an estimated requirement of 70 µg/d. Vitamin K deficiency occurs during fat malabsorption of which gallbladder stones is a common cause. Vitamin K is routinely administered prior to operations on the gallbladder to decrease this risk of haemorrhage. Antagonists of vitamin K such as warfarin are used as anticoagulants in the treatment of prothrombotic conditions.

Vitamin K is routinely administered to newborn children to prevent haemorrhagic disease

7.4.3.1 Metabolic role of vitamin K

Vitamin K is required for the post-translational modification of several glycoproteins. It is responsible for the conversion of glutamyl residues into gamma-carboxyglutamyl residues (Figure 7.6). These residues help the protein to bind to membrane surfaces. It is believed that gamma-carboxyglutamic acid residues strongly chelate calcium, and positively-charged calcium forms ion bridges to negatively-charged phosphate head groups of membrane

• **Figure 7.6** Role of vitamin K in the post-translational modification of proteins

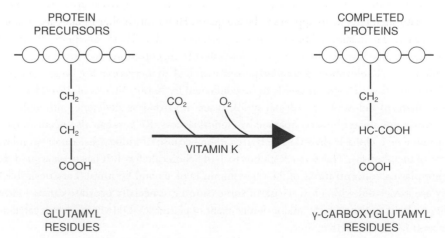

phospholipids. The first proteins to be identified were those in the clotting cascade and include prothrombin, factor VII, factor IX and factor X. Proteins C, S and Z which are modulators of the procoagulant pathway were later identified as being vitamin K-dependent along with osteocalcin and matrix Gla protein in bone which are involved in bone mineralization.

■ 7.4.4 VITAMIN E

Vitamin E was first discovered as a factor essential for normal reproduction in rats. Vitamin E is an antioxidant and consists of a family of related tocols and tocotrienols of which the most abundant are alpha-tocopherol and gamma-tocopherol. The richest dietary sources are vegetable oils, especially sunflower oil, and most of the vitamin E in the UK diet is derived from margarines and cooking oils. Nuts and wholemeal cereals are also rich sources. Deficiency of vitamin E is regarded as iatrogenic (i.e. caused by human intervention) and results in increased rates of lipid oxidation. This can result in anaemia from the haemolysis of erythrocytes as a consequence of lipid peroxidation, the accumulation of oxidized lipoprotein pigment (lipofuscin) in adipose tissue, myopathy (muscle damage) and neuropathy. A metabolic form of vitamin E deficiency occurs in abetalipoproteinemia, a rare genetic defect resulting in the lack of apolipoprotein B which is necessary for the transport of vitamin E in plasma.

7.4.4.1 Metabolic role of vitamin E

Vitamin E is located in membrane lipids and acts to protect polyunsaturated fatty acids in membrane lipids from damage by free radicals. Vitamin E is a chain breaking antioxidant. Its ring structure with methyl groups enables it to form a stable free radical which can be regenerated, possibly involving a reaction with vitamin C. Free radicals are continually generated during metabolism and a complex set of antioxidant defences are present to ensure that they are contained. The first line of defence involves metalloenzymes such as selenium-containing glutathione peroxidase, zinc-containing catalase, and copper, zinc and managanese-containing superoxide dismutases. The consequences of selenium and vitamin E deficiency in experimental animals share some similarities and both are exacerbated by a high intake of polyunsaturated fatty acids. The requirement for vitamin E increases with increasing intakes of these and an intake of 0.4 mg RRR-alpha-tocopherol/g polyunsaturated fatty acids appears to be adequate. However, higher intakes are required if polyunsaturated fatty acids with five and six double bonds, as found in fish oil, are consumed.

Vitamin E is a fat-soluble antioxidant

Vitamin E is transported on plasma LDLs and plasma concentrations are normally expressed having been adjusted for plasma cholesterol concentrations. Normal values for alpha-tocopherol are greater than 2.25 μmol/mmol cholesterol.

It has been argued that an increased intake of vitamin E may decrease the risk of cardiovascular disease and ageing by decreasing oxidative damage. However, large randomized controlled trials of vitamin E supplementation show neither harm nor benefit. Vitamin E is relatively non-toxic in amounts up to 1 g/d. There is no UK RNI but the US RDA is 10 mg RRR-alpha-tocopherol equivalents/d (15 iu/d). Median intakes in the UK are estimated to be 9.3 mg alpha-tocopherol equivalent/d for men and 6.7 mg/d for women.

SUMMARY

- Vitamins are organic substances which the body requires in small amounts for its metabolism, but which it cannot make for itself in sufficient quantities.
- Thiamin functions as a coenzyme in the pyruvate dehydrogenase reaction. Deficiency affects the nervous system, resulting in the disease beri-beri.
- Coenzymes derived from niacin act as redox carriers. Niacin deficiency causes the disease pellagra, which is associated with maize-based diets.
- Coenzymes derived from riboflavin act as redox carriers. Riboflavin deficiency is widespread but not generally fatal.
- Deficiencies of biotin and pantothenic acid are rare.
- Vitamin B_6 is a coenzyme for transamination reactions. Recommended intakes are related to protein intake.
- Vitamin B_{12} and folate are involved in one carbon transfer reactions and nucleic acid synthesis. Deficiency causes megaloblastic anaemia.
- Vitamin C can be synthesized by most other species except primates. It acts as a water-soluble antioxidant and facilitates several hydroxylation reactions.
- Vitamin A functions in the visual cycle and also has a role in regulating growth and cell differentiation.
- Vitamin D can be synthesized in the skin when exposed to sunlight. It functions in the control of calcium homeostasis.
- Vitamin K functions in the coagulation pathway.
- Vitamin E is a fat-soluble antioxidant. Requirements are related to polyunsaturated fatty acid intake.

FURTHER READING

Bender, D.A. (1992) *Nutritional Biochemistry of the Vitamins*. Cambridge: Cambridge University Press.
Institute of Medicine (2000) *Dietary Reference Intakes for Thiamin, Riboflavin, Niacin, Vitamin B$_6$, Folate, Vitamin B$_{12}$, Pantothenic Acid and Choline*. Washington: National Academy of Sciences.

DEFICIENCY AND TOXICITY DISORDERS

■ 8.1 INTRODUCTION

Nutritional deficiencies occur for a variety of reasons such as an inadequate supply or variety of foods in the diet or because disease processes interfere with the absorption and metabolism of nutrients. Some deficiencies are regarded as iatrogenic, that is they are caused artificially by human intervention. Protein energy malnutrition (PEM) is the term used to describe the consequences resulting from an intake of food that is insufficient to meet energy requirements. It is usually accompanied by a deficit in several micronutrients. Those most at risk from PEM are children under the age of 5-years-old living in the less economically developed countries. The combination of infectious diseases such as diarrhoea and measles with PEM results in a high proportion of children dying before the age of five years in these countries. In the economically developed countries, PEM is rarely seen in children but is encountered in hospital patients with chronic diseases such as cancer and alcoholism and in patients with psychiatric disorders such as anorexia nervosa.

Deficiencies of four minerals (iodine, iron, selenium and zinc) are known to cause diseases in humans of which the most prevalent are iron and iodine. As shall be discussed, iodine deficiency is globally the most important cause of brain damage during pregnancy and can easily be prevented. Iron deficiency resulting in anaemia particularly affects women of reproductive age in both developed and developing countries. In the case of iodine and selenium deficiency diseases, the cause is a lack of the mineral in the soil rather than a faulty diet. The causes of iron and zinc deficiencies are complex and depend to a large extent on the bioavailability of the mineral in the diet.

With regard to vitamin deficiency diseases only those of vitamin A, thiamin, riboflavin, niacin, folate and vitamin B_{12} result in widespread public health problems. With the exception of rickets and osteomalacia, whose causation is complex, deficiencies of the remaining vitamins are rare or iatrogenic. As discussed previously, vitamin deficiencies are much more likely to occur where there is a lack of dietary diversity and consequently it is not surprising that vitamin deficiency diseases caused by a lack of the vitamin in the diet are uncommon in the UK where there is a superabundance of food from a wide range of sources.

Currently, there is some concern regarding the potential adverse effects resulting from the overconsumption of some vitamins, especially of retinol, vitamin D and vitamin B_6. Minerals can also be toxic if consumed in excess, particularly in the case of iron, zinc, selenium, iodine and fluoride. However, more significant are toxicities caused by heavy metals. This chapter describes the causes and consequences of the major deficiency and toxicity disorders.

■ 8.2 PROTEIN ENERGY MALNUTRITION

In third world situations by far the most vulnerable group is young children, and the effect of inadequate nutrition is to slow or stop their growth, so measurement of growth rate is a very sensitive indicator of nutritional status. When the malnutrition becomes more severe, or when the people affected are adults, then there will be a net loss of body tissue. Thus the clearest manifestation of PEM is a deficit in the child's height or weight when compared with standard values for children of the same age. The severity of malnutrition is classified by the degree of stunting (low height for age) or wasting (low weight for height) (see Box 8.1). It appears that chronic malnutrition slows growth, and

---

BOX 8.1 CLASSIFICATION OF MALNUTRITION

There are many ways of classifying children according to the severity of malnutrition, but the system that is now recommended by the World Health Organisation is based on standard deviation scores, commonly known as z-scores. These are calculated by comparing the height and weight of the malnourished child with the heights and weights of a reference population of well-nourished American children. The National Center for Health Statistics (NCHS) has data from measurements made on thousands of children at each age. Thus the distribution of heights of well-nourished children of a particular age can be plotted, and the median and standard deviation of this sample can be calculated. The height of a malnourished child of the same age is then compared with the median, and the difference from the median is expressed as a multiple of the standard deviation to give the child's height for age z-score. The child's weight for height z-score is calculated in the same way.

	Mild	Moderate	Severe
STUNTING HEIGHT FOR AGE Z SCORE	−1 to −2	−2 to −3	< −3
WASTING WEIGHT FOR HEIGHT Z SCORE	−1 to −2	−2 to −3	< −3

Example:

For boys aged 2.0 years the median height is 86 cm and the standard deviation is 6 cm. Thus if a 2-year-old boy is found to have a height of 77 cm, it can be calculated that this is 9 cm below the median height for age, or $9/6 = 1.5$ standard deviations below the median. Hence the boy's height for age z-score is −1.5, and he is considered to be mildly stunted.

causes stunting, whereas acute episodes cause loss of weight from a reasonably well-grown body, and thus wasting. There may also be situations where stunting is caused by a diet that supplies adequate amounts of energy but insufficient protein, but this is probably quite rare.

The most extreme cases of stunting and wasting are called marasmus, where there is virtually a complete loss of subcutaneous fat, and the skin hangs in loose folds. The head looks big in proportion to the body, the eyes may look wide and staring. A very different picture may result when there is a more sudden, acute bout of malnutrition, giving the syndrome that is known classically as kwashiorkor. The most obvious feature is oedema, up to 30 per cent of body weight may be additional extracellular fluid. This is entirely interstitial, as plasma volume is usually decreased. Hepatomegaly and fatty liver are also usually found, as are skin changes known as crazy-paving dermatosis, with areas where dried skin peels off to leave pale, unpigmented areas. The hair comes out easily, and sometimes areas of it change colour (the so-called flag sign).

Marasmus and kwashiorkor are extreme forms of PEM, but far more children are affected by moderate degrees of stunting and wasting

The normal adaptive response to low food intake is for basal metabolic rate to decrease to minimize the negative energy balance. Part of this is achieved by changes in body composition. Fat reserves are used up to provide fuel, and lean tissue is lost to minimize the number of cells requiring energy. Muscle is lost, which may not have any immediate consequences except that the child becomes less active, ultimately appearing apathetic. It stops playing and exploring its environment, and psychomotor development is retarded. In adults the person becomes less able to work and ultimately to find food. The loss of respiratory muscle leaves the person vulnerable to respiratory infections. Skin is lost, and becomes more easily damaged and less effective as a barrier against infections and parasites. Quite a lot of the smooth muscle of the intestine is lost quite quickly. This affects the body's ability to absorb nutrients when it is refed. It also affects the ability of the gut to act as a barrier to infectious organisms.

There may also be a loss of highly metabolically active tissues such as the liver, heart and kidney. Many people who live on chronically low intakes show such changes in body composition, and this appears to be a useful adaptation which allows them to maintain energy balance, but the functional consequences become apparent when these small organs are affected by disease and are unable to respond because they have no reserve capacity. There is some evidence that brain growth is affected by malnutrition, but it tends to be much better protected than most other organs. As far as mental function is concerned, it remains controversial as to whether there is any direct effect of malnutrition on mental development.

There is also some evidence of a decrease in energy expenditure per cell. One of the major components of basal metabolism is the sodium potassium ATPase. A reduction in sodium pump activity will save energy, but at the expense of accumulating sodium intracellularly and losing potassium from cells. These changes will affect enzyme activities, and will have to be reversed when the patient is refed. Another process that can use a lot of energy is temperature regulation. Malnourished people become less able to keep warm or keep cool, and this is a particular problem when there is an infection.

Many studies have reported changes in hormone levels in malnourished people. Insulin tends to be low and cortisol high, causing some insulin resistance probably mediated by high plasma NEFA concentrations (see Chapter 9). Growth hormone levels tend to be high, mobilizing fat and glucose, but IGF levels are low so no growth is achieved and no protein is deposited. Thyroid hormone levels are also low, keeping metabolic rate low also.

It is well known that malnutrition damages immune function. This includes the afore-mentioned effects on the barrier functions of the gut and the skin and the decrease in respiratory muscle function. There is also atrophy of the thymus, spleen and lymph nodes, and a reduction in the number of circulating T-lymphocytes. On the other hand, humoral immunity tends not to be badly affected. Numbers of B-lymphocytes are relatively normal, as are most immunoglobulin levels, indeed IgA levels may be modestly elevated, as one might expect in people who are likely to be chronically infected. Reduced immune function makes it more likely that people will be infected, and each infection will have more severe effects. Gastrointestinal infections are particularly common, causing diarrhoea which decreases nutrient absorption and increases losses. Respiratory infections are also very common, increasing energy requirements and further weakening the individual. There is thus a vicious circle of infection and malnutrition, with each contributing to the other.

The consequences of infectious diseases in malnourished people are much more severe than in well-nourished people; diseases such as measles can be devastating. How-ever, PEM usually coexists with micronutrient deficiencies, particularly of vitamin A. Thus although most of the deaths of children in malnourished communities are recorded as being due to an infectious disease, in reality malnutrition is a major contributory cause.

The dietary cause of PEM is the consumption of too little food. This not usually because insufficient food is available (with the exception of droughts causing localized famines in remote areas) but because many people do not have access to it, for political, social or economic reasons (e.g. civil war, landless labourers). There are also a number of theories about the effects of the qualitative aspects of diet composition on the differ-ent manifestations of PEM, for example the difference between kwashiorkor and marasmus. One popular theory was that marasmus was caused by a lack of energy in the diet while kwashiorkor was caused by a lack of protein. The idea was that the lack of protein in the diet causes the liver to be unable to synthesize export proteins. Thus serum albumin levels decrease and so fluid is retained, and the inability to synthesize apolipoproteins means that lipoproteins are not secreted from the liver. This causes lipid to be deposited in the liver, making it enlarge and become fatty. However, biochemical investigations failed to support this idea. For example the oedema was found not to be due to low serum albumin. It is now known that low serum albumin is part of the acute phase response to infection. Analysis of the diets of children with marasmus and kwashiorkor showed that the ratio of protein to energy was quite similar in both conditions. Consequently, it cannot be simply that children with kwashiorkor are eating enough energy but not enough protein.

Other theories about the dietary causes of marasmus and kwashiorkor include the involvement of toxins, such as aflatoxin, or the role of other nutrient deficiencies, such as a lack of antioxidants allowing free radical damage to impair liver metabolism. It was argued that aflatoxins form free radicals that are hepatoxic and are not readily broken down in malnourished children. Such factors clearly may contribute to the pathology but are not the primary cause. It is most likely that the manifestation of PEM seen in any particular child results from a combination of diet and infections, and the extent to which the particular child is able to adapt metabolically. Chronic low intake and low grade

A vicious cycle of malnutrition and infection contribute to high childhood mortality rates in developing countries

infections may lead to stunting and ultimately marasmus, whereas an acute decrease in food intake, perhaps associated with a more severe bout of diarrhoeal disease may precipitate kwashiorkor. Breast feeding and the age of weaning are also important. Breast milk contains a number of factors which inhibit bacterial growth, such as lysozyme, lactoferrin and secretory IgA. Moreover, even a moderately malnourished mother continues to secrete reasonable quantities of breast milk. Bottle feeds, in contrast, may be made up with contaminated water, leading to a high incidence of diarrhoea, or they may be made up too dilute. Similarly when the child is weaned the weaning food may be too dilute, so that the child simply cannot consume a large enough volume to satisfy its requirements for either energy or protein.

■ 8.3 VITAMIN A DEFICIENCY DISEASE

The term vitamin A deficiency disease (VADD) is used to describe the consequence of a lack of vitamin A. It has superseded the term **xerophthalmia** which was previously used to describe the ocular signs of vitamin A deficiency which can result in visual impairment and even blindness. It is now recognized that vitamin A helps maintain normal immune function and children with suboptimal intakes are at an increased risk of death from infectious diseases such as measles. Children between the ages of 6 months and 6 years living in developing countries, particularly those of sub-Saharan Africa, the Indian sub-continent and South East Asia, are most at risk of developing VADD. This is a major contributor to childhood mortality and a major cause of blindness in those countries. The Sight and Life Organisation estimates that 200 to 300 million children are at risk of vitamin A deficiency, and an estimated 3 million children are clinically affected. Every year, 500,000 of these children go blind, most of them dying within one year. The reasons why VADD is prevalent are that the intake of fat is low, which means that β-carotene is poorly absorbed; there is a lack of dietary diversity; and infectious intestinal disease is prevalent, which also interferes with the absorption of β-carotene.

The earliest sign of VADD is a decreased plasma concentration of retinol ($< 20 \, \mu g/dl$). This then results in abnormal cell division (metaplasia) which can affect cell-mediated immunity and the epithelial tissues of the respiratory and digestive tract, making them more susceptible to infection. This subclinical phase of deficiency is then superseded by observable clinical changes in the deficiency disorder that is generally referred to as **xerophthalmia**. The first sign is nightblindness (**nyctalopia**) which is an inability to see under conditions of low light intensity. This is a result of an inadequate supply of retinol to the rods which is required for the formation of 11-*cis*-retinal which forms part of the visual pigment rhodopsin. The next stage progresses to signs seen in the outer eye where there is a generalized drying up of the mucous membranes on the conjunctiva and the invasion of the conjunctiva by capillaries. The conjunctiva takes on a wrinkled appearance near the cornea, which appears dull instead of shiny. This process is called **xerosis** (drying up) and is accompanied by the deposition of keratin plaques on the eye derived from undifferentiated columnar epithelial cells. Sometimes spots called Bitot's spots are seen on the conjunctiva; these have a foamy appearance (Figure 8.1). If as few as 1 per cent of children show clinical signs of vitamin A deficiency in a population, it is likely that a far greater number will have low serum concentrations of retinol which puts them at an increased risk of death from infectious diseases.

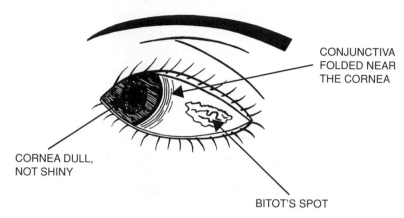

• **Figure 8.1** Ocular signs of vitamin A deficiency

CONJUNCTIVA
FOLDED NEAR
THE CORNEA

CORNEA DULL,
NOT SHINY

BITOT'S SPOT

These early stages of VADD are reversible if promptly treated with vitamin A, which is usually administered in large doses (20,000 μg retinol palmitate/d for two days by mouth or by intramuscular injection of a water-soluble emulsion in the presence of malabsorption or vomiting). If untreated, the disorder progresses to cause keratomalacia which results in permanent scarring and irreversible blindness in the affected eye. In developing countries it has been possible to reduce the incidence of VADD by the administration of prophylactic doses of 66,000 μg of vitamin A palmitate in oil orally, once every 3 to 6 months to children aged 1 to 4 years old; the dose is halved for those < 1 year. This policy of massive oral supplementation has not only reduced the incidence of xerophthalmia but has led to significant reductions in childhood mortality from measles and other infectious diseases. In the longer term, diversification of diet and improved hygiene are necessary to prevent VADD. The diet should include dark green leafy vegetables, carrots and yellow fruits, such as mango and papaw. In developed countries, a substantial contribution is made by full-fat dairy products to the intake of vitamin A and this is why low fat dairy foods are not generally recommended for children below the age of five years.

■ 8.4 RICKETS AND OSTEOMALACIA

Prior to 1900, about two-thirds of infants in the UK were affected by rickets and it was known as the English disease. The residents of industrial towns lived under clouds of black smoke from the burning of soft coal, with the result that the ultraviolet rays of the sun were largely screened out and were insufficient to produce vitamin D. Another factor that increased risk was prolonged breastfeeding as breast milk is a poor source of vitamin D. The incidence of rickets declined dramatically from the 1920s onwards. In part this can be attributed to better living conditions but also to changes in diet. Cod-liver oil was widely used as a supplement and it was government policy to administer it to young children during the Second World War and into the 1950s. Another major factor for the decline in rickets was the increase in calcium intake, mainly from milk products, and the decline in the consumption of cereals high in phytate such as oats in Scotland and Ireland, and unleavened wheat flour. Rickets is now uncommon among the white populations of the UK although occasional cases are seen among some vegetarian groups, particularly Rastafarians and Hindus. Rickets still remains a major public health problem in Middle Eastern countries and in urban China where in the 1980s it affected on average 40 per cent of all children under 3 years of age.

The characteristic signs of rickets are a protruding abdomen, beaded ribs (the so-called 'rachitic rosary'), bowed legs, knock knees, cranial bossing (thickening of parts of the skull), pigeon chest (the breastbone or sternum is pushed backwards as it descends, forming a depression between the ribs) and an enlargement of the epiphyses. The epiphyses are the regions at the ends of the long bones which are separated from the shaft of the bone, or diaphysis, by a layer of cartilage called the epiphyseal plate. These regions are mineralized during growth and eventually become part of the shaft of the bone. Teeth may erupt in an abnormal manner and the enamel may be defective. Malformed pelvic bones in women cause serious difficulties in childbirth. Permanent crippling results if severe cases are not treated. Other abnormalities associated with rickets are flabby muscles, and muscle spasms (in severe cases). The deformities of rickets (curving and twisting of the bones from their normal shape) are most likely to be found in the bones that bear the most weight or stress, such as the leg bones.

The cause of rickets is complex and is not simply a consequence of low exposure to sunlight but also low availability of calcium from the diet caused by phytic acid. In the 1960s and 70s rickets re-emerged as a public health problem in the Asian community in the UK. Anti-nutrients such as phytic acid and dietary fibre, particularly in chapattis (unleavened breads), appear to have been implicated in 'Asian rickets', and reducing dietary phytic acid promoted healing. It also appears that rickets is far more prevalent in parts of the world where exposure to sunshine is high e.g. in the Middle East and Pakistan. In these countries unleavened bread which is high in phytate is commonly consumed. In Holland, rickets was found to affect between one quarter and a half of infants brought up on a macrobiotic diet. As expected, the prevalence of rickets was lower in the summer months and the high rates of rickets was attributed to the absence of dairy products from the diet and the presence of large amounts of phytic acid rich foods, particularly brown rice in the diet.

Rickets is caused by low absorption of calcium

Adequate exposure to sunlight or *uv*-B radiation will enable the synthesis of vitamin D. However, in Northern latitudes there is virtually no synthesis between the months of November and March. Most individuals accumulate vitamin D in the summer months that tides them through the winter months. Studies on Asians show that they accumulate less vitamin D stores than whites, probably due to different cultural practices. The wearing of dark clothing and restriction of exposure to sunlight as practised by Muslim women (e.g. wearing a burka) in many Middle Eastern countries both contribute to low vitamin D stores. Supplementation of the diets of infants over 6 months with vitamin D is advised. This is more important for breastfed infants than formula fed infants, where the formula is fortified. Many commercial weaning foods are fortified, as are common foods like breakfast cereals.

It is difficult to obtain accurate figures on the incidence of osteomalacia in the population, but it appears to be more common in the elderly population than previously realized. The National Dietary and Nutritional Survey of people aged 65 years and over found that approximately 98 per cent had vitamin D intakes below the recommended level of 10 µg per day and a large proportion also had low plasma concentrations of 25-OH vitamin D, particularly those living in institutions, as they had little exposure to sunlight. However, avoiding a diet rich in phytates appears to be central to the prevention of rickets and osteomalacia coupled with an adequate intake of calcium from dairy foods such as milk, cheese and yoghurt.

■ 8.5 PELLAGRA

Pellagra is a deficiency disease that is primarily a consequence of an inadequate intake of niacin and/or tryptophan. It is endemic in some parts of Southern Africa where maize is the staple food. Pellagra is associated with maize-based diets because the niacin in maize is in the form of niacytin which is unavailable for absorption in the human gut (this also applies to most other cereals as well) and the main protein in maize, zein, is almost devoid of tryptophan. Endemic pellagra has been noted among poor peasants of the Deccan plateau of India who subsist on a staple diet of sorghum. Although this cereal contains adequate amounts of tryptophan, it contains excessive concentrations of leucine which interfere with the conversion of tryptophan to niacin.

Pellagra tends to occur in spring and early summer when food supplies are least varied, or in times of famine, drought or extreme poverty when no other food is available. It can also be induced by treatment with certain drugs (e.g. isoniazid – a drug used to treat tuberculosis) that interfere with the conversion of tryptophan to niacin, or it can develop in other cases of disturbed tryptophan metabolism (e.g. carcinoid syndrome and Hartnup disease).

Pellagra is often referred to as the deficiency of the three Ds – dermatitis, diarrhoea and dementia. It is characterized by a dermatitis (inflammation of the skin) on areas of the skin exposed to the sun. The skin on the neck, chest, and back of the hands may become brown and scaly. Initial symptoms include a smooth, red tongue, a sore mouth, and ulceration of the inside of the cheeks. The diarrhoea is caused by damage to the epithelial lining of gut, and if present is likely to cause other nutrient deficiencies. Dementia is the most serious consequence. It starts with headaches, vertigo and depression and progresses through hallucinations to delirium, convulsions and death.

> Pellagra is associated with an over-dependence on maize and is characterized by dermatitis, diarrhoea and dementia

■ 8.6 THIAMIN DEFICIENCY

The disease beri-beri has been known for thousands of years in China, but large epidemics only appeared at the end of the nineteenth century, with the advent of the mechanical milling of rice. It is caused by over-reliance on a single staple food, polished rice, and is thus relieved by increasing the variety in the diet. Thiamin (and indeed many other micronutrients) are present in the germ and aleurone layers of the rice grain and these are removed by the polishing process. Hence a diet dominated by polished rice provides large amounts of carbohydrate but not enough thiamin to metabolize it. This situation is relatively rare nowadays, but thiamin deficiency is becoming increasingly common amongst derelict alcoholics in all countries. Here it is due to a monotonous diet of alcoholic beverages, which contain little thiamin, combined with alcohol-induced damage to the intestine, affecting absorption, and to the liver, affecting phosphorylation of thiamin.

Several distinct forms of beri-beri have been described, although there are also patients who show features of more than one form. Dry beri-beri is the chronic form, and is characterized by a progressive peripheral neuropathy. This leads to muscle wasting, which is the most prominent sign. Symptoms include a burning sensation, muscle cramps and stiffness in the legs, then numbness which starts in the fingers and toes and gradually spreads centrally. Loss of motor function follows loss of sensation, and this in turn leads to muscle wasting. When this affects the respiratory muscles the patient becomes unable to cough effectively, and is thus highly vulnerable to respiratory infection, leading to pneumonia and death.

Alcoholics are at risk of thiamin deficiency

Wet beri-beri is recognized as the acute form. Peripheral oedema is the most prominent sign, and is usually accompanied by anorexia. Death may occur through heart failure, because of an inability to clear the fluid load. Acute cardiac beri-beri (shoshin) is characterized by cardiac hypertrophy and weakness in the absence of neuropathy or significant oedema. The main signs are breathlessness and palpitations. Acute infantile beri-beri causes anorexia, tenderness, oedema, then tachycardia and tachypnoea and ultimately death from heart failure. A large proportion of the victims of the large-scale outbreaks of beri-beri in the late nineteenth century were infants. Typically they were being breastfed by a mother with marginal thiamin status who may have shown no signs of deficiency herself, but her breast milk thiamin content would be low and the baby's high metabolic rate makes its thiamin requirement per unit energy intake rather higher than the adult's.

Thiamin deficiency has also been identified as the cause of the Wernicke-Korsakoff syndrome. Wernicke's encephalopathy involves nystagmus (rapid, jerky eye movements), confusion, muscle weakness and ataxia, giddiness and anorexia. It can be rapidly reversed by thiamin injections, but may progress to an irreversible stage, Korsakoff's psychosis. Here the sufferer is unable to form new memories, and may try to hide this by making up wild stories (confabulation).

■ 8.7 IODINE DEFICIENCY DISEASE

Iodine deficiency disease (IDD) is the term used to describe the consequences of an inadequate intake of iodine which include goitre, endemic deaf mutism, endemic cretinism and Keshan-Beck disease (a form of arthritis). Globally it is estimated that 1.6 billion people are at risk of iodine deficiency; it affects 50 million children and 100,000 cretins are born annually.

Endemic IDD occurs where the dietary intake is less than 20 μg/d. Affected areas tend to be isolated, limestone or mountainous areas such as the Himalayas. It is rare in coastal regions because seafood is a rich source of iodine. IDD also occurs in parts of Europe, particularly Italy, but it is becoming increasingly uncommon because food sources are diverse and traded internationally so that people are no longer dependent upon locally produced food. Goitre is the most visible manifestation of IDD and it tends to affect women during their reproductive years more than men. It is characterized by an enlargement of the thyroid gland which is situated at the base of the larynx. Besides being physically unattractive it is also associated with an increased risk of developing thyroid cancer. Goitre is a physiological response of the thyroid gland to become a more effective trap of iodine which is required for the synthesis of thyroxine. The pituitry gland produces thyroid stimulating hormone (TSH) in response to low thyroxine concentrations. Elevated plasma TSH levels can be used as an indicator of the adequacy of iodine intake. Thyroxine is important in regulating metabolic rate and individuals with goitre have low metabolic rates. Adequate production of thyroxine is required for normal foetal development particularly of the nervous system. Women who have goitre are at an increased risk of giving birth to children who are deaf mutes or are cretins. Cretinism is characterized by impaired mental development and characteristic physical deformities of the face. Iodine deficiency disease is easily prevented by the iodization of salt and this is conducted in many countries. An alternative strategy has been to inject groups which are at risk with iodized oil. Intakes of iodine in healthy populations are in the range of 100–200 µg/d. The use of iodized salt provides on average 70 µg/d. In the UK, salt is generally not iodized and the RNI in the UK is set at 140 µg/d; a significant proportion of iodine is derived from milk products.

Iodine deficiency is easily prevented by iodization of salt

■ 8.8 NUTRITIONAL ANAEMIAS

Anaemia is the most prevalent nutritional disorder worldwide. It is defined in terms of haemoglobin concentrations of less than 13 g/dl in men and 11.5 g/dl in women. The most common cause of anaemia is an inadequate supply of iron in the diet. Women during their reproductive years are more at risk than men because of blood losses caused by menstruation. Iron deficiency anaemia is almost twice as prevalent in vegetarians as in omnivores. This is because plant sources of iron are less well absorbed than animal sources. Between 15–20 per cent of women aged 12–45 suffer from iron deficiency anaemia in the UK. The main symptom of anaemia is tiredness, but if severe it will result in breathlessness and pains in the legs. In developing countries the prevalence and severity of anaemia are greater. In part this is because the diet consists mainly of food of plant origin but also because of the high prevalence of infectious intestinal parasitic disease, such as hookworm and malaria.

Iron deficiency anaemia is common in women during their reproductive years

Iron deficiency anaemia results because not enough iron is available for haemoglobin formation. As a consequence red blood cells (RBC) are produced at a normal rate but are not packed full of haemoglobin. The description of the blood film is a microcytic hypochromic anaemia. RBC populations are termed **microcytic** if Mean Corpuscular Volume is less than 80 fL and **hypochromic** if Mean Corpuscular Haemoglobin is less than 27 pg/RBC. Iron deficiency anaemia is not very responsive to changes in diet, at least in the short term, and generally requires treatment with iron supplements.

Anaemia can also be caused by deficiencies of folate and/or vitamin B_{12}. In this case, the number of RBC formed is decreased and they are packed full of haemoglobin. This is called a macrocytic anaemia and the Mean Corpuscular Volume is > 95fL. However, it is not possible to classify an anaemia precisely from examining the blood film. If a bone marrow biopsy is conducted megalobasts will be seen, this is why these anaemias are called megaloblastic. Megaloblastic anaemia can occur in late pregnancy as a consequence of folate deficiency. It can also occur because of a combination of dietary vitamin B_{12} and folate deficiency, especially in vegetarians of South Asian ethnic origin.

Pernicious anaemia is a term used to describe the megaloblastic anaemia resulting from a failure to absorb vitamin B_{12} and this is the most common form of megaloblastic anaemia encountered in the UK. Patients have to be treated with regular injections of vitamin B_{12} every 6 weeks or so. If they are given folic acid, it cures the anaemia and allows the more insidious neurological symptoms of vitamin B_{12} deficiency to progress. In order to distinguish between deficiencies of folate and vitamin B_{12}, the concentrations in blood can be measured.

■ 8.9 TOXICITIES

Because small amounts of nutrients are essential, it does not necessarily follow that more is better: in some cases they are acutely toxic. In this section, the molecular basis for the toxicity of certain vitamins and minerals is discussed.

■ 8.9.1 VITAMIN TOXICITIES

Vitamins A, D and B$_6$ are regarded as toxic when consumed in excess. The toxicity of the remaining vitamins is low.

8.9.1.1 Vitamin A

Symptoms of acute vitamin A toxicity include abdominal pain, anorexia, vomiting, blurred vision, irritability and headache. It was first reported among Arctic explorers who ate polar bear's or seal's liver. Acute toxicity has also been reported in infants given vitamin supplements where it causes an increase in intracranial pressure resulting in bulging of the fontanelles. In adults toxicity is usually a consequence of an intake of 100,000 µg RE (retinol equivalent). Infants below the age of 6 months have been shown to develop acute symptoms following a single dose of 7,500–15,000 µg RE, whereas a dose of 30,000 µg RE appears to be well-tolerated in older infants. In vitamin A toxicity, fasting plasma levels are elevated up to 2,000 µg/dL (normal values are 20–80 µg/dL).

> Vitamin A in the form of retinol is toxic and can cause birth defects with intakes in excess of 3,000 µg RE/d and may increase the risk of hip fractures

Chronic toxicity of retinol in adults is generally attributed to supplemental doses of greater than 7,500–15,000 µg RE/d, over weeks, months or years. Symptoms of chronic toxicity include dry thickening of the skin, cracking of lips, conjunctivitis, erythematous eruption, alopecia, reduced bone mineral density, bone joint pain, chronic headache, intracranial hypertension and hepatotoxicity. However, there is some evidence that more moderate intakes of vitamin A in excess of 3,000 µg RE/d increase the risk of hip fracture in older women.

It is known that the synthetic retinoid etretinate causes birth defects and it is believed that this effect is mediated through the retinoic acid receptors on HOX genes. Animal studies have found that high intakes of retinol are teratogenic. Some, but not all studies have found a relationship between high intakes of retinol and birth defects. However, the relationship appears stronger for retinol supplements than for dietary sources. It has been shown that retinol supplements are more rapidly oxidized to retinoic acid following ingestion. Retinol in food is more likely to be transported postprandially as retinyl esters in chylomicrons as opposed to retinol in supplements which may be transported directly to the liver in the hepatic portal vein.

β-carotene in contrast is relatively non-toxic and is not associated with any of the symptoms described above. An excessive intake does, however, turn the skin yellow (*xanthosis cutis*) but this appears to be of no pathological significance. Several trials have investigated the effects of high intakes (20 mg/d) of β-carotene on the risk of cancer and cardiovascular disease. In two studies in groups at high risk of lung cancer (smokers and asbestos workers) the risk of cancer was increased. However, carotene supplementation had no adverse effects in lower risk groups.

It has been suggested that the upper safe limit for retinol intake should be no more than 3,000 µg RE/d. A safe upper level of intake of β-carotene of 7 mg/d has been suggested for supplements. However, this is not applicable to vegetable sources where the biovailability of β-carotene is only about 30 per cent of that in supplements.

8.9.1.2 Vitamin D

Excessive vitamin D intake may lead to hypercalcaemia (high blood calcium concentrations) and hypercalciuria (increased calcium excretion). Vitamin D toxicity results in the deposition of calcium in soft tissues and eventually causes kidney damage. It can easily be diagnosed by measuring plasma 25-OH vitamin D levels which are elevated as much as fifteenfold. Toxicity is generally only seen with intakes in excess of 250 µg/d. There clearly are genetic disorders where infants show signs of vitamin D toxicity with lower intakes (idiopathic hypercalcaemia). Such children have a characteristic elfin face, are mentally retarded and have supravalvular aortic stenosis. It has been argued that intakes of 25–50 µg/d of vitamin D may enhance renal stone formation in susceptible individuals, but the evidence is not convincing because this level of intake does not lead to elevations of plasma 25-OH vitamin concentrations beyond that obtained by exposure of the skin to UV radiation. Few foods, with the possible exception of oily fish and fish liver, supply sufficient amounts to result in toxic effects. Consequently, toxicity invariably results from the excessive intake of vitamin D from supplementary sources. An upper safe limit of 25 µg/d from supplementary sources has been suggested. However, this appears to be on the conservative side in view of the experimental evidence.

8.9.1.3 Vitamin B₆

Long-term use of pyridoxine (generally in excess of 50 mg/d) can result in peripheral neuropathy which appears to be reversible if the use of the supplement is ceased in time. Large doses of pyridoxine (2–3 g/d) can cause permanent nerve damage. Symptoms include tingling in the hands and feet, a stumbling gait, numbness around the mouth, a characteristic 'stocking-glove' sensory loss and lack of muscle coordination. A satisfactory explanation for the toxicity of pyridoxine has yet to be advanced. A safe upper limit of 10 mg/d has been suggested.

■ 8.9.2 MINERALS

Virtually all minerals are poisonous in excess and their toxicity depends to a large extent on their solubility. For example, potassium and sodium salts are relatively toxic compared with calcium salts. In practical terms, toxicities of iron and the heavy metals are of the greatest significance.

8.9.2.1 Potassium

Potassium chloride can cause cardiac arrest if taken in high doses that are rapidly absorbed. Consequently, pharmaceutical preparations of potassium chloride are designed to release potassium slowly. An excessive intake of potassium from food can also cause gastrointestinal symptoms characterized by abdominal pain, nausea and vomiting. This can happen if prodigious quantities of apples or bananas are consumed too rapidly. In chronic renal failure the capacity of the kidney to excrete potassium may be impaired and life-threatening hyperkalaemia can occur, in which case it may be necessary to restrict the intake of potassium.

8.9.2.2 Iron

Excess iron is toxic, causing vomiting, diarrhoea, and damage to the intestines and liver. Most cases of acute iron poisoning occur in children, due to accidental ingestion of iron supplements intended for their mothers. The toxicity of iron depends upon the form in which it is present. Ferrous ions are absorbed more efficiently than ferric ions. The acute toxic dose of iron in infants is considered to be approximately 20 mg/kg body weight, associated with gastrointestinal irritation, whilst systemic effects do not generally occur at doses < 60 mg/kg bw. The lethal dose in children is approximately 200–300 mg/kg bw. Prescription iron supplements typically contain about 50 mg iron usually as ferrous sulphate or gluconate.

Iron within the body is transported by iron binding proteins that prevent it interacting with cellular components. In iron toxicity, this capacity for binding iron is exceeded and free iron is able to catalyse the Fenton reaction which converts the superoxide radical $O_2^{\cdot}$ and hydrogen peroxide to the hydroxyl radical $OH^{\cdot}$ which is a potent reactive oxygen species capable of causing free radical damage to cell membranes, proteins and DNA. Free radical damage stimulates fibrosis and causes scarring of the liver.

Iron is toxic in the body when it is not bound to proteins because it catalyses the Fenton reaction leading to the generation of the hydroxyl radical

Accidental iron poisoning in adults is rare. However, haemochromatosis is a relatively common disorder where the regulation of iron absorption is disturbed so that even moderate intakes of iron accumulate in the body. It affects around one in three hundred of the population and the gene for haemochromatosis is carried by 1–2 per cent of the population. The excess of body iron accumulates first in the liver and later in other organs, resulting in liver damage and other clinical disorders. Liver disease is characterized by progressive fibrosis leading to cirrhosis and liver cancer. The harmful effects can be completely prevented, and life expectancy can be restored to normal, if the disease is detected early, before the development of cirrhosis, and treated by phlebotomy (blood letting).

8.9.2.3 Heavy metals

Lead, cadmium and mercury are heavy metals naturally present in the environment but also as a consequence of pollution (e.g. from lead-containing paint, batteries, plumbing, industrial emissions and leaded petrol). They are present at low concentrations in most foods, with environmental sources being the main routes of contamination. Lead, cadmium and mercury have no known beneficial biological effects and long-term (chronic) exposure can be harmful.

8.9.2.4 Lead

Lead (Pb) absorption may constitute a serious risk to public health. It is a cumulative poison, which may cause reduced cognitive development and intellectual performance in children and increased blood pressure and cardiovascular diseases in adults. Childhood lead poisoning usually occurs through the inadvertent consumption of lead. Over the past 20 years, childhood lead poisoning has declined dramatically in the UK and USA due to limits on lead in petrol, paint, food cans, and other consumer products such as pencils. The main sources of exposure are now from dust from lead-containing paints and lead from the domestic water supply. The water supply can acquire lead from lead plumbing particularly in soft water areas where the pH of the water is low, thus allowing the lead to dissolve in the water. In old houses, lead can still leach into the water supply and this is why it is advised never to take water for drinking from the hot water supply but only from the mains. Lead was also used for the capsules on bottles of wine and crystals of lead tartrate sometimes form on the cork. Lead capsules are now being replaced with plastic capsules. Besides having adverse effects on the nervous system, lead is a bone-seeking mineral and accumulates in bones and teeth. Archaeologicalists have found that the Romans had high levels of lead in their bones and some have speculated that this may have come from lead piping and could even have been responsible for the decline of the Roman Empire. Recent research has suggested that when lead is incorporated into tooth enamel the teeth are more prone to caries. It is also possible to measure past exposure by determining the levels in teeth. Lead also interferes with the synthesis of porphyrins which are the building blocks of haemoglobin, and chronic lead poisoning results in anaemia. Normal plasma lead levels are below 0.5 μmol/l; levels above 1 μmol/l are a cause for concern. Average dietary exposure of the UK population to lead (0.026 mg/d) is well below the tolerable daily intake of 0.21 mg/d. However, cases of lead poisoning are still reported in the population and it is often difficult to trace the source.

8.9.2.5 Cadmium

Cadmium is mainly used for electroplating, galvanization processes and in batteries. Cadmium compounds have varying degrees of solubility ranging from very soluble to nearly insoluble, which affects the extent to which they are absorbed and hence their toxicity. Cadmium is a cumulative contaminant, which accumulates in the kidney causing damage that eventually results in high blood pressure and an increased risk of related disorders such as stroke; cadmium may also increase risk of cancer. High cadmium levels have been found in vegetation near smelting works and fungi in particular accumulate heavy metals and so are good biosensors. In areas of Japan and China where rice is grown on soils contaminated by mining wastes, people have suffered adverse health effects from cadmium intake. This is associated with a crippling condition, 'itai-itai' (ouch-ouch) disease which is characterized by pain in the back and joints, osteomalacia, bone fractures, and occasional renal failure. Some areas of the UK have high levels of cadmium in their soil (e.g. Shipham in Somerset) and this leads to high levels in home grown vegetables but this does not seem to be associated with adverse health consequences. The effects of cadmium toxicity appear to be more severe in populations with poor intakes of iron, calcium and zinc. Cadmium can also accumulate in the liver and kidney of livestock that graze on pastures where soil levels are high in it. Average dietary exposure of the UK population to cadmium is 0.012 mg/day compared with a tolerable daily intake of 0.06 mg/day.

8.9.2.6 Mercury

Mercury compounds are neurotoxins, which may induce alterations in the normal development of the brain in infants and at higher levels may induce neurological changes in adults. Mercuric chloride, which was at one time used to blacken top hats and formerly resulted in madness in hatmakers (hence the phrase 'mad as a hatter'), is very toxic with as little as 100 mg causing poisoning and 500 mg being fatal. However, mercury amalgam which is used in dental fillings is non-toxic. Organic forms of mercury such as methyl mercury are more toxic than metallic or inorganic forms due to their greater ease in crossing the blood-brain barrier. The mechanism by which mercury ultimately causes nerve damage is uncertain. Mercury is known to form adducts across the double bonds of polyunsaturated fatty acids that make up the synaptic membranes and it also impairs the synthesis of ADP-dependent proteins in neurons. These organic forms, such as methyl mercury, can accumulate in the marine food chain and cause poisoning in people who consume contaminated fish. This is illustrated by the experience of fishermen who developed neurological symptoms and paralysis in Minamata, Japan where there was a smelting works discharging large amounts of mercury salts into the sea. Average dietary exposures of the UK population to mercury (0.003 mg/day) are well within the recommended safe levels of exposure of 0.3 mg/week. However, as high levels of mercury (on average 1.5 mg/kg) have also been found in shark, marlin and swordfish, women are advised to avoid these fish during pregnancy.

Heavy metals Pb, Cd and Hg are cumulatively toxic. Pregnant women should avoid eating shark, marlin and swordfish

SUMMARY

- Protein energy malnutrition, vitamin A deficiency, goitre and the nutritional anaemias are the major nutritional deficiencies occurring in developing countries.
- Rickets and osteomalacia result from a combination of an inadequate supply of vitamin D and low availability of calcium from the diet.
- The main cause of vitamin B_{12} deficiency is a failure to absorb the vitamin and this results in pernicious anaemia.
- Iron deficiency anaemia is the most common nutritional deficiency in the UK and mainly affects women during their reproductive years.
- Excessive intakes of retinol, vitamin D and vitamin B_6 are toxic.
- Iron overload most commonly results from a genetic disorder called haemochromatosis.
- Heavy metals (Pb, Cd and Mg) are significant toxicity diseases.

FURTHER READING

McClaren, D.S. and Frigg, M. (1997) *Sight and Life Manual on Vitamin A Deficiency Disorders (VADD)*. Basel: Sight and Life Organisation.

McLaren, D.S. (1992) '*Colour atlas and text of diet-related disorders*', in *Nutritional Disorders*. London: Wolfe Medical Press.

Vieth, R., Chan, P.R. and MacFarlane, G.R. (2001) 'Efficacy and safety of vitamin D_3 exceeding the lowest observed effect level', *Am. J. Clin. Nutr*, 73: 288–94.

9

DIET-RELATED DISEASE

In the economically developed areas of the world, food shortage and nutritional deficiencies are uncommon but diet plays a major role in the causation of several non-communicable diseases such as cardiovascular disease, diabetes mellitus, cancer and dental caries. These diseases are sometimes referred to as diseases of affluence. Overweight and obesity may contribute to their causation but these disorders are also prevalent in people who are not overweight. Unlike simple nutritional deficiencies, these disorders are caused by a combination of factors, some constitutional and others environmental.

Much of the evidence for the role of diet in the causation of non-communicable disease is derived from epidemiological studies. These can broadly be divided into 1) ecological studies, where the patterns of disease and food intake are compared between different populations or countries, and 2) cohort studies, where a well-defined group of people is followed up for the incidence of new diseases or events. The major weakness of ecological studies is that they are unable to control for lifestyle differences and genetic factors between communities. Cohort studies are more powerful because statistical adjustments allow estimates of the contribution to risk made by many factors. The most powerful type of study is the prospective cohort study, where measurements of exposure are made prior to the occurrence of disease. Risk of disease is usually described in terms of relative risk. This is normally calculated either by reference to a group unexposed to the risk factor or by reference to subjects in the bottom third (tertile) or fifth (quintile) of the distribution (the reference category is assigned a relative risk of 1). Dose response relationships can be compared by determining whether risk increases with exposure. For example, in a study of alcohol intake and risk of cirrhosis of the liver, the relative risk was 4.0 among subjects consuming four or more drinks/d compared with non-drinkers but there was no increased risk in people who drank fewer, up to one drink/d (Figure 9.1). It is important that relative risk should not be confused with absolute risk. For example, the relative risk of dying suddenly is greater for younger men who are obese that that for older men but the absolute risk is very much greater for older men.

• **Figure 9.1** Relationship between alcohol intake and relative risk of cirrhosis of the liver in men (*Source*: Thun *et al.*, 1997)

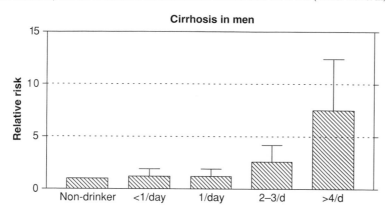

Epidemiological studies often yield conflicting results for a variety of reasons: different population groups, different sample sizes, different methods of ascertainment of end-points and confounding factors. A technique called systematic review is often used to pool the results of studies to provide a more robust answer. This process sets down rules for inclusion of studies in the review, so that poorly designed or described studies are excluded. The data from the selected studies are then pooled and a statistical technique called meta-analysis is conducted to calculate the statistical significance of the pooled results. Systematic reviews are regarded as giving the most reliable answer when a large number of studies have been conducted but they tend to be over conservative where only a few studies have been conducted. For example, many studies have examined the effect of lowering blood pressure on the risk of coronary heart disease and some studies showed a significant effect while others failed to find a significant effect. A systematic review of the trials by Collins *et al.* from the MRC Clinical Trials Unit, Oxford concluded that lowering diastolic blood pressure by about 5 mm Hg decreased the risk of CHD by 14 per cent.

Epidemiological studies can show associations and identify risk factors but can never prove a causal association. In order for associations to be convincing there should be consistency in the findings, strength of association, a dose response relationship and a plausible biological mechanism. In the case of the association of alcohol with cirrhosis of the liver discussed above, this is plausible because alcohol is metabolized in the liver and excess alcohol is known to cause a fatty liver, which can in turn cause cirrhosis. Confounding is the term used to describe a statistical association which is not causally related. For example, several studies have noted a lower risk of lung cancer among vegetarians than omnivores. However, the vegetarians are predominantly non-smokers so the association between vegetarianism and lung cancer is confounded by a difference in lifestyle (i.e. smoking). In order to prove causality it is often necessary to put the question to test in a randomized controlled trial. However, with some diseases such as cancer and heart disease this is very difficult as they develop over a period of 20–30 years and dietary patterns can change with time. In this chapter, we discuss the hazards posed by diet-related diseases and the molecular basis for the role of dietary constituents in the causation of obesity and diabetes, cardiovascular disease, cancer and dental caries.

■ 9.1 OBESITY

■ 9.1.1 DEFINITIONS AND PREVALENCE

Obesity can be defined as an excessive accumulation of body fat. Women are naturally fatter than men and so the definitions of obesity in terms of body fatness differ between men and women. For example, the body of a healthy man would typically contain 10–15 per cent by weight fat, whereas that of a healthy woman would be between 20–30 per cent fat.

In practice it is not very convenient to measure body fatness (although a number of devices are marketed that estimate body fat based on bioelectrical impedance) and obesity is usually defined in terms of body weight. The Quetelet or body mass index (BMI), which is the body weight in kg divided by the square of height in metres, is a convenient tool for estimating what proportion of the population is obese.

$$BMI = \frac{\text{weight in kg}}{\text{height in m}^2}$$

Under weight BMI <18 kg/m^2; normal 18–24.9 kg/m^2; overweight 25–29.9 kg/m^2; obese >30 kg/m^2; morbidly obese >40 kg/m^2

Overweight may or may not be due to increases in body fat. As muscle is more dense than fat it is possible to misclassify individuals as obese when they are muscle bound and contain a very low level of body fat (for example body builders). The cut off points for BMI are different for children because their body proportions change with growth.

In 2001, the proportion of UK adults who have a BMI >30 kg/m^2 was about 18 per cent of the population. This has increased markedly since twenty years ago when less than 6 per cent fell into this category. In the USA, the situation is worse with over 20 per cent of the population having a BMI >30 kg/m^2 and a significant proportion with a BMI >40 kg/m^2.

■ 9.1.2 PREVENTION OF OBESITY

Obesity is a consequence of an imbalance between energy intake and expenditure. There is considerable concern about the increasing prevalence of obesity worldwide, especially among adolescents. The evidence that decreased energy expenditure resulting from decreased physical activity is the primary cause of this increase is overwhelming. There is no evidence to suggest that total energy or fat intakes have increased. Indeed in the UK, they have declined by almost a third over the past forty years. There is much debate as to whether a low fat:carbohydrate ratio decreases the population risk of obesity. In the normal situation there is very little synthesis of fat from carbohydrate so most adipose tissue is derived from dietary fat when energy requirements are exceeded. Advocates of low fat/high carbohydrate diets claim that energy intakes are likely to be lower than on high fat diets because of differences of energy density. However, soft drinks and alcoholic drinks such as beer can also contribute substantially to total energy intake.

■ 9.1.3 TREATMENT OF OBESITY

There are few effective treatments for obesity. Although obesity can be treated by decreasing energy intake, most patients regain their weight on cessation of dieting. The major difficulty is bringing about a long-term change in behaviour. Behavioural therapy coupled with a nutritionally balanced reduced energy intake is probably the safest way to treat obesity providing there is compliance to the treatment. Exercise, while important for preventing weight gain and improving insulin sensitivity, is not an effective means of losing weight. Surgical interventions including jaw wiring, surgical removal of fat, liposuction and modification of the gastrointestinal tract all have hazards associated with their use and so are only appropriate in extreme cases. For example, banded gastroplasty, which is a surgical procedure where the size of the stomach is reduced, has been shown to improve survival in morbidly obese patients. Various slimming drugs have been developed but these are generally not effective alone without a reduction in food energy intake. Appetite suppressant drugs which were related to amphetamines (e.g. fenfluramine) have now been withdrawn because they cause undesirable side-effects such as valvular heart disease and pulmonary hypertension. Sibutramine is a new appetite suppressant drug that works by blocking the reuptake of neurotransmitters and appears to be effective. However, it is unsuitable for use by people with psychiatric disorders and has some unpleasant side-effects (headache and insomnia). One of the few drugs shown to be safe and moderately effective is the lipase inhibitor orlistat, which is used in conjunction with dietary advice to follow a very low fat diet. If the subject consumes too much fat it results in fatty diarrhoea and "anal leakage".

■ 9.1.4 HEALTH RISKS OF OBESITY

The health risks vary according to 1) the degree of obesity; 2) age; 3) other lifestyle factors such as physical activity and smoking; and 4) the pattern of fatness. The male 'apple' shaped pattern is more harmful than the female 'pear' shaped pattern, for reasons that appear to be related to the action of insulin, as discussed below. Data collected by life insurance companies show that very fat men are more likely to die suddenly under the age of 40 years. However, the relationship between BMI and mortality is more complex in older people and follows a J-shaped curve (Figure 9.2). In order to estimate the health risks of obesity, it is necessary to exclude smokers. This is because smokers are lighter in weight than non-smokers but have a very greatly increased risk of premature mortality. Individuals who are underweight are at increased risk of dying prematurely and there is a nadir between 22–26 kg/m^2. As BMI increases above 28 kg/m^2 mortality increases exponentially. Individuals who smoke are at higher risk across the range of BMI but the risk to health of smoking is greater than that of obesity so that a thin smoker is more likely to die prematurely than an obese non-smoker. Although the relative risk of death associated with obesity is greater in young people, the absolute risk is greater in older people and underweight is associated with a greater risk of premature mortality than overweight. Analysis of the causes of death show that an increased BMI results in a greater risk of death from diabetes, cardiovascular disease and some forms of cancer.

Morbidity (illness) is also increased with obesity: for example, there is an increased risk of osteoarthritis, caused by increased wear and tear on joints, gallbladder disease, varicose veins and reproductive problems in women. However, there are some benefits

The health risk of obesity depends upon the extent of obesity and in absolute terms is greater in older people

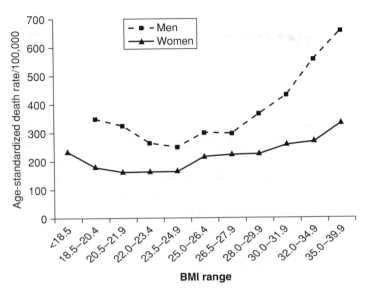

• **Figure 9.2** Age-adjusted mortality rates in middle-aged non-smoking adults (*Source*: Calle *et al.* (1999) *N. Eng. J. Med.* 341: 1097–1105.)

Obesity increases the risk of Type II diabetes, stroke, coronary heart disease, some cancers, osteoarthritis and varicose veins

of plumpness (BMI 24–27 kg/m^2) particularly in older women as it is associated with a lower risk of osteoporosis. In extremely obese people (BMI >40), life can be threatened by sleep apnoea (cessation of breathing) and a tracheotomy may be necessary to prevent sudden death. Estimates of the BMI associated with a 20 per cent and 50 per cent increased risk of all causes of mortality according to age and gender, compared with individuals with a BMI of 21 kg/m^2 are shown in Table 9.1.

Obesity does not affect the risk of Type I diabetes, which is caused by a failure of the pancreas to secrete insulin. However, obesity, along with low physical activity, is a major cause of Type II diabetes. Type II diabetes results from a failure of tissues to respond to insulin and it is the most common form of diabetes in middle-aged and elderly people (it used to be called maturity-onset diabetes). While there clearly are genetic components that determine susceptibility to Type II diabetes (for example, people of South Asian origin and Pima Indians are known to be at increased risk), the disorder becomes more prevalent with increasing obesity.

Table 9.1 Body mass indices (BMI) associated with a 20% and 50% increase in mortality from all causes compared to subjects with a BMI of 21 kg/m^2 in non-smokers

Age	Men		Women	
	20%	50%	20%	50%
30–44	23.8	27.2	26.0	32.1
45–54	24.2	28.1	24.8	29.4
55–64	24.7	29.1	25.9	32.0
65–74	28.2	37.0	29.9	40.8

Source: Stevans *et al.* (1998) *N. Eng. J. Med.* 331: 1–7.

Diabetes is probably the greatest hazard associated with moderate obesity because of the long-term damage it causes to the cardiovascular system, kidneys and eyes. The risk of diabetes increases exponentially with increasing BMI. Indeed most individuals with a BMI greater than 35 will become diabetic. The risk of insulin resistance, which is an underlying pathology in the causation of diabetes and cardiovascular disease, also increases with increasing BMI. In the next section the metabolic basis for the relationship between obesity, insulin resistance and diabetes will be discussed.

■ 9.2 TYPE II DIABETES

This form of diabetes is probably a consequence of inappropriate storage of fat in tissues such as muscle and liver which impairs the action of insulin. The consequence of a lack of the action of insulin is that blood glucose concentrations rise. This deprives tissues of glucose and in the longer term glucose can react with proteins to cause the formation of glycosylated proteins that can lead to damage to the microcirculation, particularly in the retina, kidney and nervous system. To compensate for the lack of effect of insulin, the body produces more insulin and high levels of insulin in the blood have damaging effects on the circulatory system, itself resulting in raised blood pressure and damage to the vascular endothelium (an early event in atherosclerosis).

Many people are not aware that they have Type II diabetes until it becomes severe. The presenting symptoms are usually tiredness, excessive thirst and frequent urination. If the concentration of blood glucose exceeds the renal threshold, glucose will spill over into the urine and so diabetes can be diagnosed by measuring glucose in the urine. However, a more accurate test is to measure the fasting plasma glucose concentration which should be below 7 mmol/l.

A high proportion of Type II diabetes goes undiagnosed and can cause long-term damage to the cardiovascular system

About 2–3 per cent of the UK middle-aged population have Type II diabetes and in the USA the prevalence is higher, about 6 per cent. At least twice as many people have impaired glucose tolerance, a condition that usually precedes Type II diabetes. Impaired glucose tolerance can be determined by measuring the change in blood glucose concentration following a standard 75 g glucose load. In the normal state, plasma glucose concentration will rise to a peak approximately 45 mins following the glucose load and then fall back to fasting value by 2 h. In subjects with glucose intolerance, plasma glucose will remain elevated at 2 h. Plasma insulin concentrations are greatly elevated in subjects with glucose intolerance following a glucose load, which indicates that there is resistance to the action of insulin.

Insulin resistance, which is defined as resistance to the glucoregulatory actions of insulin, is now believed to be the underlying cause of Type II diabetes and also contributes directly to causing cardiovascular disease. A fundamental consequence of insulin resistance is that fasting and postprandial concentrations of insulin in the blood are elevated. Insulin resistance prevents the inhibition of lipolysis as well as the uptake of glucose by cells. Insulin resistance is characterized by the accumulation of visceral fat and is accompanied by a number of metabolic abnormalities (hypertension, Type IV hyperlipidaemia, gout and decreased fibrinolytic activity) that all confer increased risk of cardiovascular disease. This is sometimes referred to as syndrome X or metabolic syndrome but the term insulin resistance syndrome is preferred.

Insulin resistance is the key feature predisposing to and causing Type II diabetes

In a normal healthy subject, the release of fatty acids from adipose tissue is inhibited by insulin following a carbohydrate containing meal. Where there is insulin resistance, insulin fails to inhibit lipolysis which means that the release of fatty acids from adipose tissue remains uncontrolled and plasma concentrations of non-esterified fatty acids (NEFA) are increased. This has two major effects. Firstly, the elevated NEFA concentrations stimulate triacylglycerol (TAG) synthesis within the liver and the secretion of TAG-rich very low density lipoproteins (VLDLs). Prolonged elevations of plasma TAG results in a fall in plasma high density lipoprotein (HDL) concentration and an increase in the concentration of small, dense low density lipoproteins (LDLs) by the action of cholesterol ester transfer protein (CETP). CETP exchanges cholesteryl esters in exchange for TAG and the resulting TAG enriched LDLs and HDLs become substrates for hepatic lipase which decreases their density. Secondly, elevated NEFA further aggravates insulin resistance because of their inhibitory effects on both glucose transport and glucose metabolism in skeletal muscle. Elevated plasma concentrations of insulin also result in an increase in blood pressure probably by increasing sympathetic nervous system activity and by causing damage to the vascular system.

A major new development has been the recognition that adipose tissue is not an inert organ but produces chemical mediators such as leptin, acylation-stimulating protein (ASP) and adiponectin. Leptin acts as a physiological signal to decrease appetite and increase energy expenditure. Patients with leptin deficiency become obese at an early age, primarily from an insatiable appetite. Treatment of such children with leptin results in decreased appetite and weight loss. Leptin production is mainly regulated by insulin-induced changes of adipocyte metabolism and plasma leptin concentrations are higher in obese subjects than lean subjects.

ASP increases the efficiency of triacylglycerol synthesis in adipocytes from TAG-rich lipoproteins such as chylomicrons and VLDL. Effective fatty acid trapping by adipose tissue may prevent some of the undesirable effects resulting from elevated plasma NEFA concentrations. Adiponectin increases insulin sensitivity in adipose tissue and its production is stimulated by agonists of peroxisome proliferator-activated receptor-gamma (PPARγ). Plasma levels of adiponectin have been found to be lower in obese people who go on to develop diabetes.

As mentioned previously, there is some evidence to suggest that it is the inability to store fat in appropriate sites that causes insulin resistance. Lipodystrophies are characterized by selective but variable loss of body fat with the consequences that fat is stored in muscles and the liver. Lipodystrophies have become increasingly important as they can result from the use of anti-viral drugs used to treat patients with HIV. Patients with lipodystrophies exhibit many of the metabolic abnormalities associated with insulin resistance even though they are not obese.

It seems that visceral fat within the abdominal cavity plays an important role in insulin resistance. With increasing obesity, the size of abdominal fat stores increases. Fat stored within the abdominal cavity appears to be a greater contributor to plasma NEFA than fat stored elsewhere. This may also explain why the 'apple' pattern of obesity is more strongly associated with insulin resistance than the female 'pear' shape pattern. The visceral fat pool which is typically 4–5 kg is the first to be mobilized. It has been observed that sensitivity to insulin increases as this pool is reduced. Several trials have shown that it is

Insulin resistance results in raised blood pressure, low HDL and small dense LDL which increase risk of heart disease

possible to prevent overweight and obese individuals who are glucose intolerant from developing diabetes by losing moderate amounts of weight (5 kg) and taking regular exercise (e.g. brisk walking for about 30 mins daily).

■ 9.3 CARDIOVASCULAR DISEASE

Cerebrovascular disease (stroke) and coronary heart disease (CHD) are leading causes of death worldwide. The risk of both is greater in men than women and increases greatly with age. Stroke is defined by the WHO as 'Rapidly developing clinical signs of focal (or global) disturbances of cerebral function, with symptoms lasting 24 h or longer or leading to death, with no apparent cause other than of vascular origin'. Stroke can result either from the rupture of an artery (cerebral haemorrhage) or blockage of an artery supplying the brain (cerebral infarction). The incidence of stroke resulting from cerebral haemorrhage is strongly linked to raised blood pressure. CHD results from the blockage of one of the coronary arteries supplying the heart muscle and this results in a heart attack which is characterized by severe chest pain (angina) and damage to the heart muscle (myocardial infarction). Cerebral infarction and CHD share a common pathology which is atherosclerosis of the large arteries.

Atherosclerosis is a process by which nodular cholesterol enriched plaques are laid down in the intima of large to medium arteries. This is a chronic process that develops silently over 20–30 years. Rupture of an atherosclerotic plaque triggering the formation

Atherosclerosis is a major risk factor for coronary heart disease and occlusive stroke and develops over a 20–30 year period

• **Figure 9.3** Relationship of atherosclerosis with coronary heart disease and stroke

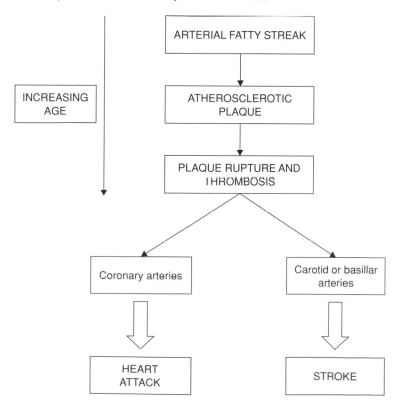

of a blood clot (thrombosis) that blocks an artery is the pathological process that leads to a clinical event. The tissue supplied by the artery is starved of oxygenated blood and dies. Coronary thrombosis is the main cause of a heart attack and a thrombosis in a carotid or basilar artery is usually the cause of cerebral infarction. Prevention of CHD and stroke is more important than treatment as a high proportion of first heart attacks and strokes are fatal and occur without warning.

Epidemiological studies show that raised blood pressure is the single most important risk factor for stroke. Numerous risk factors for CHD have been identified which can be subdivided into those that are unalterable, such as age, gender and heredity, and those that can be modified, such as diet, exercise and smoking. Diet influences the risk of CHD in several ways but most attention has focused on the effects of diet on blood pressure and plasma cholesterol concentrations. Risk of CHD increases across the entire range of plasma cholesterol concentrations but when it is greater than 5 mmol/l its adverse effects are amplified by high blood pressure and cigarette smoking. A population's risk of CHD is strongly associated with the average cholesterol concentration. Although the Japanese population has a high rate of smoking and high blood pressure compared with the UK and other Northern European countries, their rates of CHD are low. This has led to the view that elevated plasma cholesterol is the single most important risk factor in determining a population's risk of CHD. However, within the UK where most middle-aged men and women have raised blood cholesterol, cigarette smoking is the most important predictor of risk. Moderate alcohol intake up to 21 units/week in women and 28 units/week in men is associated with a reduced risk of CHD (1 unit = 10 ml ethanol and is equivalent to a small glass of wine, $^1/_2$ pint of beer, or a single shot of spirits). The mechanism by which protection is afforded is not understood. However, heavy alcohol consumption is associated with increased risk of stroke and CHD. The other major dietary factor shown to influence CHD risk is the intake of oily fish which appears to protect against fatal CHD. It is believed that long chain $n-3$ fatty acids afford protection by decreasing the susceptibility of the heart to cardiac arrhythmias.

Lowering plasma cholesterol decreases the incidence of heart disease whereas lowering blood pressure mainly reduces the incidence of stroke and to a lesser extent that of CHD. In the next sections we shall consider the molecular mechanisms by which dietary intake influences blood pressure and plasma cholesterol concentrations.

■ 9.3.1 BLOOD PRESSURE

Normal blood pressure is defined as 120/80 mm Hg (the first figure represents the systolic blood pressure and the second figure the diastolic blood pressure). Hypertension is defined as a blood pressure in excess of 140/90 mm Hg. Severe hypertension is defined as a blood pressure in excess of 160/105 mm Hg. Blood pressure increases with age and tends to be higher in men than women until the menopause, when it rises in women. Blood pressure is a function of cardiac output and peripheral resistance in small arteries. The main cause of hypertension is increased peripheral resistance. Epidemiological studies have found high blood pressure to be positively associated with BMI, sodium and alcohol intakes and negatively associated with potassium intake.

In communities where the intake of salt is low, the increase in blood pressure with age is less marked. This suggests that the effect of salt (sodium chloride) is greater in

High blood pressure is the major risk factor for haemorrhagic and occlusive stroke

Elevated plasma cholesterol is the major factor determining a population's risk of CHD

middle age and beyond. Randomized controlled trials have shown that decreasing the intake of salt results in a fall of about 5–10 mm Hg in systolic blood pressure in subjects who are hypertensive or over the age of 50 years. However, a reduction in salt intake in normotensive subjects has little effect and may even slightly increase blood pressure. The difference in response probably reflects differences in the activity of the renin-angiotensin system between young, when it is active, and older people, where it may be less active. An increased intake of potassium in the form of fruit, vegetables and lean meat results in a fall in blood pressure of between 2–5 mm Hg. However, the blood pressure lowering effects of potassium are lower on a low salt diet. Potassium helps stimulate sodium excretion by increasing aldosterone secretion. The major target of aldosterone is the distal tubule of the kidney, where it stimulates the exchange of sodium and potassium. Sodium balance can then be maintained at a lower perfusion pressure. However, the exact mechanism whereby potassium lowers blood pressure is uncertain.

The risk of developing hypertension increases with overweight and obesity and is probably a consequence of insulin resistance as discussed previously. Weight loss of about 5 per cent body weight usually results in a 3 mm fall in both systolic and diastolic blood pressure. Heavy alcohol intakes (more than 21 units/week for women and 28 units/week for men) are a cause of raised blood pressure. The mechanism by which alcohol intake increases blood pressure is uncertain but the effects are reversible on stopping drinking. It is uncertain why alcohol increases blood pressure but it may be a rebound response to the withdrawal of alcohol which is a potent vasodilator and diuretic. Alcohol acutely suppresses vasopressin secretion and this is why it has a diuretic effect but this is followed by an increase in plasma renin concentration. However, moderate alcohol intake (1–3 drinks per week) is associated with a slight reduction of blood pressure, probably because it helps people relax.

Blood pressure is positively associated with BMI, salt and alcohol intake and negatively associated with potassium intake

■ 9.3.2 PLASMA CHOLESTEROL

Blood lipids are transported bound to lipoproteins which are classified according to their density. In fasting blood there are three major lipoproteins: very low density lipoprotein (VLDL), low density lipoprotein (LDL) and high density lipoprotein (HDL). In the fed state there are in addition chylomicrons and intermediate density lipoproteins (IDL). Cholesterol, cholesteryl esters, triacylglycerols (TAG) and phospholipids are the major lipids transported on lipoproteins. The apoproteins associated with the lipoproteins play a key role in the metabolism of lipoproteins by activating enzymes and acting as ligands for receptors (Figure 9.4). Cholesterol is required for the synthesis of membranes and steroid hormones and is transported to tissues mainly on LDL. About a quarter of the cholesterol in plasma is carried by HDL. HDL is involved in the transport of cholesterol from cell membranes in tissues back to the liver. It also plays a key role in the exchange of apolipoproteins and cholesteryl esters. The role of VLDL is to transport endogenous TAG synthesized within the liver to muscle and adipose tissue. LDLs are formed by progressive removal of lipid from VLDL (Figure 9.4).

VLDL is secreted by the liver and acquires apolipoprotein C (from HDL) which activates lipoprotein lipase located on endothelial cells. This catalyses the hydrolysis of TAG on the VLDL to release fatty acids which are then taken up by endothelial cells and transported into muscle and adipose tissue. The lipid-depleted particle is termed

• **Figure 9.4** Endogenous pathway of lipoprotein metabolism

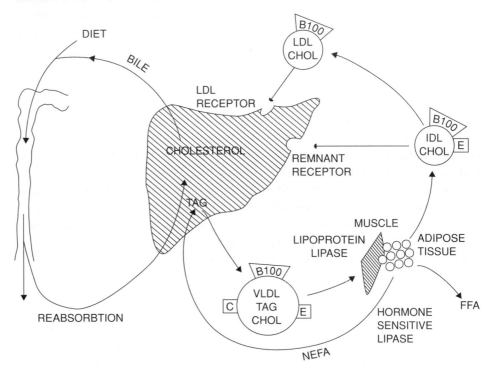

intermediate density lipoprotein (IDL). It contains two proteins – apolipoprotein E and apolipoprotein B100 (as opposed to apolipoprotein B48 in chylomicrons). Apolipoprotein E binds to a high affinity receptor in the liver which results in the uptake of the remnant particle. However, not all IDL contains apolipoprotein E and it becomes a substrate for hepatic lipase in the formation of LDL. LDL is enriched in cholesteryl ester and apoprotein B100. LDL is recognized by receptors to apolipoprotein B100, which are located mainly in the liver, and is taken up by a process of receptor mediated endocytosis. In this process, LDL is internalized and undergoes lysosomal hydrolysis to release the cholesterol. This in turn triggers three regulatory actions: 1) the synthesis of cholesterol is suppressed; 2) the excess cholesterol is converted to cholesteryl esters for storage; and 3) the synthesis of LDL receptors is decreased.

The significance of the LDL receptor in regulating plasma cholesterol concentrations was elucidated by the study of familial hypercholesterolaemia (FH) which is an inherited disorder that results in premature atherosclerosis and cardiovascular disease. Patients with FH lack LDL receptors, have extremely high plasma cholesterol concentrations and usually die from heart disease when young. Plasma cholesterol concentration fell markedly in a patient with FH who was given a liver transplant from a donor with normal cholesterol concentrations. This demonstrates the importance of hepatic LDL receptors in regulating plasma cholesterol. The homozygous form of FH is very rare but the heterozygous form is relatively common (1:500). However, the extent to which plasma cholesterol in patients with heterozygous FH is elevated is dependent on the background diet. For example, in rural China, where BMI is low and the intake of fat is low, plasma cholesterol levels are around 6 mmol/l, as opposed to 12 mmol/l among patients with FH in Hong Kong, where BMI is higher and the intake of fat is greater. Another form of FH which is equally common results from defective apolipoprotein B which is unable to bind to the LDL receptor. However, FH only accounts for about 1:250 cases of raised cholesterol.

Apolipoprotein E, a constituent of chylomicrons, VLDL and HDL, acts as a ligand for the LDL receptor and is required for hepatic uptake of IDL and chylomicrons. The gene coding for apolipoprotein E has three common alleles: ε2, ε3 and ε4, which code for three common isoforms of apolipoprotein E. Fifty-five to sixty per cent of the population are estimated to be homozygous for the ε3 allele and about 25–30 per cent carry the ε4 allele. Individuals carrying the ε4 allele have higher plasma cholesterol concentrations than those with the ε3 and those carrying the ε2 allele have the lowest concentrations and may be more susceptible to the effects of dietary saturated fatty acids and cholesterol. This apolipoprotein E polymorphism may account for up to 7 per cent of the variation of LDL and total cholesterol within a population. However, in the UK almost 80 per cent of middle-aged men have moderate elevations in blood cholesterol (>5 mmol/l) and diet is the main cause.

9.3.2.1 How high levels of plasma cholesterol cause CHD

Cholesterol crystals are found in atherosclerotic plaques and these have been shown to originate from circulating lipoproteins, mainly LDL. The cholesterol deposits are derived from dead 'foam cells', which are lipid-laden macrophages that have become trapped in the sub-endothelial space. Foam cell formation is regarded as an early step in the atherosclerotic process. Foam cells are formed from the uptake of LDL by tissue macrophages (a type of cell found in tissues which is derived from circulating monocytes). Native LDL is not recognized by macrophages as the normal LDL receptor is switched off. However, if the conformation of apolipoprotein B is modified by oxidation or glycation it is recognized by a scavenger receptor and is avidly taken up by macrophages. Modification of LDL is, therefore, a key step in foam cell formation. The oxidative modification of LDL is believed to occur in the sub-endothelial space that forms when plasma concentrations are high and is probably catalysed by enzymes expressed by endothelial and white blood cells. This is a normal physiological process whereby cellular debris is removed by macrophages and in the normal course of events this would not be harmful. However, if there is excessive foam cell formation fatty streaks occur in the artery wall and these can progress to more complex atherosclerotic lesions. Experimentally, lowering LDL cholesterol concentrations has been shown to result in a slowing and even regression in the growth of atherosclerotic plaques.

High plasma cholesterol reflects high levels of LDL. Oxidized LDL is taken up by macrophages to form foam cells that constitute the initial atherosclerotic lesion

9.3.2.2 How diet causes elevated plasma cholesterol concentrations

Plasma cholesterol concentrations depend on 1) the rate of synthesis of LDL from VLDL and 2) the activity of the hepatic LDL receptors. The main stimulus for VLDL secretion is the plasma concentration of NEFA, which is elevated in insulin resistance, and during stress. The activity of the LDL receptor is determined by a combination of genetic and hormonal factors. Certain steroid hormones increase the synthesis of LDL receptors (e.g. oestrogen and thyroid hormone) whereas others suppress their activity (e.g. corticosteroids). Plasma cholesterol rises in women after the menopause because of the lack of oestrogen. Hormone replacement therapy with oestrogen decreases LDL cholesterol and increases the receptor mediated clearance of LDL. An increased intake of soy protein has been found to lower LDL cholesterol and part of this effect may be mediated by isoflavone components present in soy that have oestrogenic effects.

The activity of LDL receptors is also regulated by the cellular cholesterol concentration and if the absorption of cholesterol from the gut is high, the synthesis of LDL receptors by the liver will be reduced and the synthesis of cholesterol decreased. Consequently, the effect of dietary cholesterol on plasma cholesterol concentrations is generally small. Increasing the intake of dietary cholesterol from zero to about 400 mg/d only increases plasma cholesterol by about 2 per cent. However, there are individuals who appear to be more sensitive to the effects of dietary cholesterol and they carry the ε4 allele for apolipoprotein E. The ε2 allele, on other hand, is associated with insensitivity to dietary cholesterol. There is a report of a patient who was homozygous for the ε2 allele and consumed 25 eggs a day but had a normal plasma cholesterol concentration.

Cholesterol is secreted into the gut with bile in response to a fatty meal. Recently, it has been shown that competitively inhibiting the absorption of cholesterol from the gut with an intake of 2–3 g phytostanols/phytosterols results in a 10 per cent reduction in plasma LDL cholesterol concentrations. This is believed to lower blood cholesterol concentrations by depleting hepatic stores of cholesterol and upregulating the expression of LDL receptors. However, higher intakes of phytostanols do not lead to greater reductions because cholesterol biosynthesis is upregulated.

The intake of saturated fatty acids (C12 to C16) has a major effect on increasing the concentration of LDL in plasma. It is believed that this effect is mediated by decreasing the binding of the LDL particle to the receptor rather than decreasing the number of receptors. Decreasing the dietary intake of saturated fatty acids by 1 per cent of the energy results in a 1–2 per cent reduction in plasma total and LDL cholesterol concentrations. In the 1970s the intake of saturated fatty acids was above 20 per cent of energy intake because butter and animal fats were widely used. Nowadays average intakes of saturated fatty acids are nearer 12 per cent of energy intakes in the UK and USA as a consequence of the replacement of fats rich in saturated fatty acids with oils and spreads rich in unsaturated fatty acids. Changing from a diet obtaining 12 per cent energy from saturated fatty acids to one obtaining less than 7 per cent from this source results in a 9 per cent reduction in LDL cholesterol concentration. This dietary change in combination with the use of products containing plant stanols and sterols would be expected to achieve a reduction in LDL cholesterol of 20 per cent. Such a change would be predicted to decrease the risk of CHD by between 20 and 60 per cent.

Obesity increases LDL by stimulating VLDL synthesis and saturated fatty acids and cholesterol decrease the removal of LDL by receptors

■ 9.4 DIET AND CANCER

Cancer is defined as a malignant growth or tumour whose cells have the properties of endless replication, loss of contact inhibition, invasiveness and the ability to spread (metastasize) and whose result, if left untreated, is generally fatal. Cancer affects many tissues especially those which have a high rate of cell division. It can occur at any stage in life but becomes more common with increasing age. Although there are genetic factors that determine risk, most cancers are caused by environmental influences. For example, in a study of twins there was relatively little concordance with regard to risk of cancer (in contrast there is strong concordance with body weight and risk of Type II diabetes). Known causes of cancer include cigarette smoking, exposure to ionizing radiation, certain infections (particularly viral infections for leukaemias and liver cancer), alcohol intake, occupational exposures to certain chemicals (e.g. tar) and compounds (e.g. asbestos). It is believed that about one-third of all cancers may be related to diet. It is well known from animal studies that restriction of food intake decreases the risk of cancer. However, compounds present in food may either increase or decrease the risk of cancer.

The incidence of cancer in the UK has been increasing partly because people are living longer. However, the pattern of cancer is changing. The most common site of cancer is the skin, but, with the exception of melanoma, it is rarely fatal. The other major sites of cancer are the lung, upper digestive tract, stomach, liver, colon and rectum, breast, ovaries and uterus, prostate and brain. The lung is the leading site of cancer but the incidence has been falling in men because many have given up smoking. However, lung cancer is on the increase in women who are continuing to adopt the habit (often to remain slim). Prostate cancer is very common in older men but is generally not fatal. Colorectal cancer is probably the next most common site of cancer and its incidence has been increasing. The incidence of stomach cancer on the other hand has been steadily falling. Breast cancer is the most common cancer in women and incidence rates have risen markedly in the UK over the past 30 years.

The strongest links for diet and risk of cancer are for tumours of the gastrointestinal tract. Most of the evidence is derived from epidemiological studies and the conclusion drawn from systematic reviews of these studies is that there is consistent and convincing evidence of a relationship between the consumption of vegetables and decreased risk of cancer of the upper digestive tract, stomach, colon and rectum. Fruit intake is associated with a lower risk of stomach cancer but not colorectal cancer. The consumption of red meat and meat products is associated with an increased risk of colorectal cancer. Obesity on the other hand is associated with an increased risk of colorectal, kidney, oesophageal, endometrial and breast cancer. There are no consistent associations of fat intake with risk of cancer but there is a protective effect of physical activity on the risk of colorectal cancer. Very hot drinks are associated with increased risk of cancer of the mouth and the upper digestive tract. The intake of alcohol is strongly associated with increased risk of cancers of the upper digestive tract and liver and moderately associated with colorectal and breast cancer. Based on these findings dietary guidelines for the prevention of cancer have been drawn up by the Department of Health. These mainly focus on avoiding obesity and increasing the intake of fruit and vegetables to five portions a day.

There are three phases involved in carcinogenesis: initiation, where damage to DNA leads to a precancerous lesion; promotion, where the precancerous lesion acquires the capacity to grow and to spread; and metastasis, where the tumour can seed cells in distant organs to produce secondary tumours. There is often a long lag phase (up to 25 years) between initiation and promotion. The molecular mechanisms by which diet can influence risk of cancer are in the initiation of damage to DNA and in the promotional phase, where diet may promote the production of growth factors.

The three phases of carcinogenesis are initiation, promotion and metastases

Carcinogens are compounds that can cause cancer. Carcinogens cause characteristic mutations in DNA and it is possible to look for the fingerprint of a carcinogen in a tumour. N-nitroso compounds and some polycyclic aromatic hydrocarbons such as benzopyrene which is found in tobacco smoke are good examples of carcinogens. Carcinogens may be present naturally in food or may be formed during cooking or processing. For example, polycyclic aromatic hydrocarbons are present in barbecued foods and significant amounts of N-nitroso compounds have been found in Chinese salted fish. More recently acrylamide, which is a potential carcinogen, has been found in a wide variety of foodstuffs, particularly fried potatoes and corn chips.

These compounds cause characteristic mutations in DNA. However, mutations occur often and there are mechanisms of DNA repair and mutated cells may be destroyed by the immune system (immune surveillance). Any nutritional effects on the immune system, for instance depressed immune function caused by malnutrition, may affect a person's susceptibility to cancer.

Although there are a large number of potentially carcinogenic compounds in food, whether they result in mutations depends on how they are metabolized within the gut and within the body. Foreign compounds undergo two types of reaction termed phase 1 and phase 2 reactions. Phase 1 reactions are metabolic transformations that may involve oxidation, reduction, amination, deamination or methylation reactions and are conducted by a group of enzymes that are part of the cytochrome P450 complex. Phase 2 reactions are conjugation reactions, typically with a sugar molecule. The purpose of these reactions is to make organic compounds more polar and water-soluble so that they can be excreted. However, phase 1 reactions can activate as well as inactivate carcinogens. For example, benzopyrene can undergo metabolic activation and one of its diol epoxides (BPDE-2) is a powerful carcinogen on the basis of its binding to DNA, mutagenicity and extreme pulmonary carcinogenicity in newborn mice. Phase 1 and 2 reactions take place mainly in the liver but phase 1 reactions also occur in the gut. Sulphur containing compounds, present in cruciferous vegetables, onions and garlic, have been found to block the activation of certain carcinogens. Cruciferous vegetables contain glucosinolates that are hydrolysed by the enzyme myrosinase to give pungent smelling compounds such as sulforaphane. Sulforaphane is a potent inducer of phase 2 enzymes. It has also been suggested that certain nutrients (selenium, vitamin E, vitamin C and β-carotene) that are involved in protecting against free radical damage may decrease the risk of cancer. However, trials conducted in developed countries using dietary supplements have generally failed to show any effect.

Food may cause cancer by supplying carcinogens or by carrying infections that can cause cancer

Some cancers are associated with microbial infections that are transmitted by food and drink. For example, there is compelling evidence that repeated infection with *Helicobacter pylori* is strongly associated with the risk of stomach cancer. *H. pylori* is known to cause gastric ulcers and individuals who have a history of peptic ulcers are known to be at increase risk of stomach cancer. The incidence of both peptic ulcers and stomach cancer has decreased markedly in the UK and USA over the past fifty years. This has been attributed to improved food hygiene and the refrigeration of food as opposed to preservation by pickling and salting. On the other hand, obesity predisposes an individual to stomach acid refluxing into the oesophagus and this is associated with an increased risk of oesophageal cancer.

In many developing countries liver cancer is the leading cause of cancer and is believed to be caused by infection with the hepatitis B virus and probably the hepatitis C virus. These viruses can be transmitted sexually or by blood as well as by shellfish and water contaminated with faeces. Individuals infected with hepatitis B have a 50 per cent lifetime risk of developing liver cancer. Foods containing aflatoxins (see Chapter 10) may also increase the risk of liver cancer, particularly where hepatitis is in epidemic. Liver cancer can also occur in patients with untreated haemochromatosis, a disease caused by an inability to control iron absorption.

Obesity may promote tumours by stimulating the production of growth factors such as hormones

Diet can influence levels of hormones that can promote the growth of tumours. Breast, endometrial and ovarian cancer are strongly related to changes brought about by ovarian hormones, particularly oestrogen. Early menopause or removal of the ovaries decreases the risk of these cancers. Drugs such as tamoxifen, which antagonizes the action of oestrogen on the oestrogen receptor ORα, have been successfully used to control and prevent breast cancer but at the same time increase the risk of endometrial cancer. Hormone replacement therapy with oestrogen also increases the risk of breast cancer in postmenopausal women. Obesity also increases the risk of breast cancer in postmenopausal women. One explanation for this is that adipose tissues synthesize oestrogen from androgens. Alcohol intake has also been found to increase the risk of breast cancer even at moderate intakes of alcohol. The reasons for this association are uncertain: it could be because alcohol increases plasma oestrogen concentrations.

The risk of breast cancer is strongly related to fertility and reproductive factors. Pregnancy before the age of 23 years, prolonged breast feeding and a late age of menarche (initiation of menstruation) are all associated with decreased risk. The age of menarche is strongly determined by nutritional status and has fallen from an age of between 16–18 a hundred years ago to below 12 years of age now. Age of menarche is strongly determined by body weight and the amount of body fat. At the other end of the scale, the age of menopause has increased from around 40 years to around 50 years. Women nowadays have more menstrual cycles because of better nutrition. However, this may result in an increased risk of breast cancer. During the luteal phase of the menstrual cycle, the combination of high oestrogen and progesterone levels stimulate breast cell division. It has been argued that increased mitosis increases the probability of mutations occurring.

Observational studies made in Africa show that cancer of the colon and rectum is very uncommon among people consuming large amounts of relatively unprocessed starchy foods. In contrast, in most developed countries where the intake of unrefined starchy foods has declined significantly and is continuing to do so, the incidence of colorectal cancer is high and increasing. The rural African diet results in large bulky faeces which pass through the gut rapidly (usually in less than 24 h) whereas on a Western diet relatively small amounts of dense faeces are produced which traverse the gut more slowly (up to 72 h). It is argued that the rapid transit time and bulky faeces seen among the rural Africans decrease exposure of the gut to carcinogens. The bulky faeces and rapid transit time in the Africans are a consequence of bacterial fermentation of dietary fibre and resistant starch in the large intestine to volatile fatty acids such as acetic, propionic and butyric acid. These fatty acids lower the pH in the colon and inhibit the formation of some potential carcinogens from bile acids which are present in the colon. Fermentation also increases the bulk of faeces and decreases transit time through the gut. It has been

Colorectal cancer may be related to events concerned with fermentation in the colon

proposed that an increased intake of foods high in fibre and containing resistant starch (e.g. bananas and pasta) may help prevent colorectal cancer.

Several intervention studies of increased fibre intake have been conducted to see if it prevents the recurrence of colorectal adenoma. However, they show no benefit. In contrast, supplements of calcium have been shown to prevent recurrence of colorectal adenoma. High intakes of calcium may decrease the cancer promoting effects of bile acids in the colon.

Some epidemiological studies suggest that the consumption of red meat or meat products is associated with increased risk of colorectal cancer. This association is only seen with high intake (above 140 g/d) and it is confounded by the association with a low intake of complex carbohydrates. The production of N-nitrosocompounds is increased with the consumption of red meat but not by white meat or fish. N-nitrosocompounds are known to cause tumours in animals and alkylated DNA adducts have been found in human colon tissue.

■ 9.5 DENTAL CARIES

Rotten teeth are the signs of a disease called dental caries. Dental caries is a bacterial disease with sugar being intimately involved. Caries is caused by dental plaque which is a sticky substance composed of millions of bacteria. Dental plaque collects around and between teeth. The initiation of caries requires the presence of a significant proportion of *Steptococcus mutans* within the plaque. *S. mutans* sticks to the tooth surface, produces more acid from sugars than other bacterial types, is tolerant of an acidic environment, and produces extracellular polysaccharides from sucrose which provide a matrix for the plaque. When the proportion of *S. mutans* in plaque is in the range 2–10 per cent, an individual is at increased risk of caries. When the proportion is less than 0.1 per cent, the risk is low. Infection with *S. mutans* usually happens early in childhood by transmission

Fermentation of sugar by dental plaque bacteria results in acid production which demineralizes tooth enamel

via the mouth e.g. by kissing. Several species of *Lactobacillus*, and *Actinomyces viscosus* also contribute to causing caries because they can produce large amounts of acid. Plaque bacteria ferment sugar to organic acids (mainly lactic acid) which lower the pH and thus cause demineralization of tooth enamel.

Sugar is the best substrate but all fermentable carbohydrate can lead to acid production: the rate of fermentation of starches depends on their structure within the food matrix and their residence time within the mouth. Sugar is more cariogenic than starch, but the amount of sugar in a food does not necessarily provide a good guide to its ability to cause dimineralization of tooth enamel. For example, in the case of fruit yoghurts containing approximately 15 g sugar/100 g, the effect is negligible because of the high calcium content of the yoghurt which promotes remineralization. Sugar typically provides 10–20 per cent of the food energy in the British diet. The development of caries is driven by the frequency with which sugar is consumed rather than the total amount. It also depends on the presence of other foods. For example, the consumption of cheese following a sugar-containing meal reduces demineralization of tooth enamel and promotes remineralization.

The susceptibility of teeth to caries is modified by fluoride. The mineral of enamel – cementum and dentine – is a highly substituted calcium phosphate salt called apatite. In newly formed teeth, this apatite is rich in carbonate, has relatively little fluoride and is relatively soluble. Cycles of partial demineralization and then remineralization in a fluoride-rich environment creates apatite which has less carbonate, more fluoride and is less soluble. Fluoride-rich, low carbonate apatite is much less soluble than apatite low in fluoride. Topical application of fluoride also inhibits acid production by plaque bacteria. Fluoride in water as well as in toothpaste and oral rinses can therefore all reduce the solubility of teeth, helping to reduce caries risk. The addition of 1 mg sodium fluoride/l of drinking water markedly reduces the risk of caries. If excess amounts of fluoride are consumed, this results in slight mottling of tooth enamel.

Fluoride, cheese and saliva promote remineralization of tooth enamel

The risk of caries is also modified by saliva which helps buffer the acid produced. Chewing promotes saliva production and can promote remineralization. National dental surveys in the UK have found a high proportion of children to have dental erosion. Dental erosion of tooth substance results from the consumption of low pH foods and drinks such as fruit juice. The frequent consumption of acidic beverages and the swishing and holding habit associated with drinking have been found to be associated with increased risk.

The prevalence of dental caries has fallen dramatically in most Western European countries in children of school age. There is no evidence that this fall is related to a change in sugar consumption and it has been attributed to increased exposure to fluoride and improved oral hygiene. However, caries in children under the age of five years is still a major problem and has been linked to the frequency of consumption of sugar containing drinks (including seemingly healthy orange juice) in trainer cups. The key to preventing dental caries is good oral hygiene to prevent the build up of plaque, ensuring an adequate intake of fluoride and avoiding the frequent consumption of sugar containing snacks between meals. Chewing sugar-free gum can also promote the flow of saliva.

SUMMARY

- Diet plays a major role in the causation of cardiovascular disease, diabetes mellitus, cancer and dental caries.
- The evidence is mainly derived from ecological and cohort studies.
- Obesity increases the risk of Type II diabetes, cardiovascular disease and some types of cancer.
- The health hazards of obesity depend upon the extent of obesity, age and gender.
- Type II diabetes is caused by low physical activity and the accumulation of visceral fat and is a consequenc of insulin resistance.
- High blood pressure is the main risk factor for stroke and is increased by obesity, alcohol and salt, and lowered by potassium.
- High blood cholesterol is the major risk factor for coronary heart disease and is influenced by the intake of saturated fatty acids and obesity.
- Alcohol intake is a major cause of cancer of the upper digestive tract and liver and contributes to causing breast cancer.
- An increased intake of fruit and vegetables is associated with a lower risk of cancer but the mechanisms for protection are uncertain.
- Dental caries is a bacterial disease caused by sugar which can be prevented by good oral hygiene and avoiding the frequent consumption of sugar.

FURTHER READING

Ashwell, M. (1997) *British Nutrition Foundation: Diet and Heart Disease*. London: Chapman Hall.

Bjorntorp, P. and Brodoff, B.N. (1992) *Obesity*. Philadelphia: Lippincott.

British Nutrition Foundation (2002) *Oral health: Diet and Other Factors*, in J. Buttriss (ed.) *Adverse Reactions to Food*. London: Blackwell Scientific Press.

Cardiovascular Review Group (1994) *Committee on Medical Aspects of Food Policy: Nutritional aspects of cardiovascular disease. Department of Health Report on Health and Social Services*, 46. HMSO: London.

Collins, R., Peto, R., MacMahon, S., Merbert, P., Fiebach, N.M., Eberlein, K.A., Godwin, J., Qizilbash, N., Taylor, J.O. and Hennekens, C.H. (1990) 'Blood pressure, stroke, and coronary heart disease; Part 2: Short-term reductions in blood pressure – overview of randomized drug trials in their epidemiological context', *Lancet*, **335(8693)**: 827–38.

Department of Health (1998) *Working Group on Diet and Cancer of the Committee on Medical Aspects of Food and Nutrition Policy. Report on Health and Social Subjects*, 48: Nutritional Aspects of Diet and Cancer. London: HMSO.

International Task Force for Prevention of Coronary Heart Disease. *Coronary Heart Disease: Reducing the Risk*, http://www.chd-taskforce.com/guidelines/ (accessed 12/02/03).

Reaven, G.M. (1999) 'Insulin resistance: a chicken that has come to roost', *Ann. N.Y. Acad. Sci.*, 892: 45–57.

World Cancer Research Fund in association with the American Institute for Cancer Research (1997) *Food, Nutrition and the Prevention of Cancer: A Global Perspective*. Washington, DC: American Institute for Cancer Research.

Food intake can influence health independently of the nutritional quality of the food. A food hazard can be defined as 'A biological, chemical or physical agent in, or condition of food with the potential to cause, an adverse health effect'. These hazards include naturally occurring and artificial toxicants present in food and the harmful effects resulting from microbial contamination of foods. The hazards posed by these compounds are dependent on potency, dose, duration and timing of exposure, age, gender and health of the individual. Compounds found in staple foods or drinks present the greatest risk as they can affect the health of very large numbers of people. Some foods are harmless to most people but cause adverse reactions in a small minority, as in the case of food allergies.

Most food is now produced by large farms, traded globally, processed industrially, and sold by large-scale food retailers. This process has reduced the cost and increased the variety of food available but presents an opportunity for foodborne pathogens and toxins to infect and poison large numbers of consumers. Furthermore, the globalization of the food trade means that food can become contaminated in one country and cause outbreaks of foodborne illness in another. Modern food production has become so complex that a systematic approach is needed to identify the hazards at each point in the food chain and to take action to prevent adverse events occurring. It has also become important to be able to trace the identity of a food back to its place of production. In this chapter, the molecular basis of food hazards will be discussed along with new developments regarding functional and genetically modified foods.

■ 10.1 IDIOSYNCRATIC ADVERSE REACTIONS TO FOOD

There is some truth in the saying that one man's meat is another man's poison. Idiosyncratic adverse reactions to food are best illustrated by reference to food allergy.

Food allergy is defined as an adverse immunological response (hypersensitivity) to food. It can manifest itself in several ways by inflammation and hives on the skin, irritation of the intestinal tract leading to malabsorption, or by anaphylactic shock, where the afflicted individual can rapidly die from cardiorespiratory failure. Food allergies with acute onset of symptoms after ingestion are usually mediated by IgE, which arms tissue mast cells and blood basophils, to result in a state termed sensitization. Re-exposure to the allergen triggers the release of mediators such as histamine and leukotrienes that cause symptoms.

In a population-based study in the UK, 20 per cent of adults thought that they had a food allergy or intolerance. However, when challenged with a panel of potentially offending foods the derived overall prevalence of food allergy was 1.8 per cent. The most common allergies are to nuts, shellfish, wheat, eggs, milk and soy. The most severe allergies are to peanuts and shellfish which can result in anaphylactic shock and death. Allergy to fruits and vegetables is common but is usually not as severe and there is cross-reactivity between different allergies. Individuals who are allergic to latex are also likely to be allergic to kiwi fruit, bananas and avocado pears. Food allergy is more prevalent in children and many grow out of their allergies. However, allergies to peanuts and shellfish tend to be lifelong. In the UK products containing even traces of peanuts are now clearly labelled so that people with a peanut allergy can avoid them. Coeliac disease, which affects around 1 in 2,000 people in the UK, is a consequence of allergy to gluten, a protein found in wheat, rye, and barley. It results in malabsorption and dermatitis and is treated by following a gluten free diet. The cause of food allergy is uncertain but it is believed that the early introduction of foods other than milk in the diet may increase the risk.

There are other idiosyncratic responses to food that do not involve allergic reactions. For example, the consumption of asparagus by some individuals results in the formation of malodorous urine smelling like rotten cabbage, which probably reflects differences in the metabolism of S-methyl methionine to dimethyl sulphide. Coffee and chocolate are known to trigger migraine in some individuals; this is probably attributable to their content of methyl xanthines. Red wine is also a well known trigger of headaches in some people and this has been attributed to resveratrol, a flavonoid present in grape skin.

> Idiosyncratic reactions to food can arise because of allergens in food or differences in the metabolism of bioactive food components

■ 10.2 NATURALLY OCCURRING TOXICANTS IN FOOD

Naturally occurring toxicants are widespread in plants and include alkaloids, (e.g. caffeine, theophylline and solanine), glycosides (e.g. glucosinolates and cyanogenic glycosides), enzyme inhibitors (trypsin inhitors and ackee toxin), inhibitors of mineral absorption (oxalate and phytic acid), lectins (e.g. phytohaemagglutinins), phenolics and a variety of compounds that have structural homology with hormones and transcription factors. People in developing countries are at much greater risk from naturally occurring toxicants because they have a limited dietary repertoire, they may out of necessity eat food which would otherwise be regarded as unfit for human consumption and they may lack the resources to process it effectively into a safe form. For example, lathyrism is a disorder that causes endemic paralysis in parts of South Asia and the Middle East and is a consequence of the consumption of large amounts of the chickling vetch pea *Lathyrus sativus* that have been inadequately processed. Small amounts of the pea are habitually consumed in endemic areas but in times of food shortage and drought intakes can be high. The toxic principle is neurotoxin 3-N-oxalyl-L-2,3-diaminopropionic acid, which acts as an inhibitor of the neurotransmitter GABA and causes paralysis.

Naturally occurring toxicants pose a relatively low risk to health in developed countries because effective food processing and a varied diet restrict exposure. Cooking inactivates many of the naturally occurring toxicants in plant foods. For example, raw red kidney beans, which contain phytohaemagglutinins and trypsin inhibitors, are poisonous if consumed raw and cause severe vomiting and diarrhoea. However, these toxic compounds are destroyed during cooking in boiling water. Food processing can also decrease naturally occurring toxicants in food. Wholewheat contains quite large amounts of phytic acid, a compound that binds to divalent cations and interferes with the absorption of calcium, iron and zinc and is important in the causation of rickets. However, the leavening of bread with yeast leads to the breakdown of phytic acid.

Cooking and food processing destroy many naturally occurring toxicants

Herbal remedies and 'health foods' on sale in the USA and Europe have resulted in serious and sometimes fatal poisoning. In one report, herbal weight reducing pills containing *Stephania tetrandra* were contaminated with *Aristolochia fangchi* and caused urothelial cancer. Preparations containing ephedra alkaloids and herbal teas containing pyrrolizidine alkaloids have also caused poisoning. The pyrrolizidine alkaloids cause liver and kidney failure and are found in the leaves of plants of the Boraginaceae, Compositae, and Leguminosae families. Comfrey and ragwort are examples of plants that contain these alkaloids. There is concern that the increase in ragwort, which is known to cause poisoning in horses and sheep, could result in pyrrolizidines finding their way into honey. Indeed, it is known that toxic honey is made by bees who feed on azaleas and rhododendrons. The toxic principle grayanotoxin binds to sodium channels in cell membranes and results in dizziness, weakness, excessive perspiration, nausea, and vomiting shortly after the toxic honey is ingested but is rarely fatal.

Toxicants in wild mushrooms result in hundreds of deaths annually particularly in Eastern Europe and China. In most cases this results from confusing poisonous with edible species. The *Amanita* species and false morel are the species often implicated in cases of human poisoning. The principal toxins (amatoxins) are taken up by hepatocytes and interfere with messenger RNA synthesis, thus suppressing protein synthesis and resulting in severe acute hepatitis and often liver failure. Hydrazine derivatives (found in the false morel) have been shown to cause cancer by causing mutations in DNA.

Natural foods can contain harmful chemicals

■ 10.2.1 PLANT CONSTITUENTS WITH HORMONAL ACTIONS

Some foods of plant origin contain compounds with hormonal actions in animals. These compounds may be the evolutionary precursors of mammalian hormones. Their physiological role in plants may be to stimulate certain growth processes such as root nodule development in legumes or to provide insect resistance by inhibiting the reproduction of pests. These compounds tend to be sterols, polyphenols or terpinoids and share structural homology with mammalian hormones. In many cases the compounds occur as glycosides which confer water solubility. For example, a water-soluble form of the active form hormone vitamin D (1,25-dihydroxycholecalciferol glycoside) has been found in certain plants such as wild oats.

Several plant compounds can mimic the action of animal hormones

The hormone modulating effects of some plants are well illustrated by reference to the effects resulting from the excessive consumption of liquorice which can result in raised blood pressure and hypokalaemia (low levels of potassium in the blood). Liquorice contains the terpinoid glycorrhizic acid (GZA), which affects the metabolism of corticosteroids. After ingestion, GZA is converted to 18-β-glycyrrhetinic acid (GRA) within the gastrointestinal tract. Both GRA and especially GZA inhibit 11-β-hydroxysteroid dehydrogenase which is responsible for the conversion into cortisone. Cortisol:cortisone ratios rise when the enzyme is inhibited. Cortisol has the same binding affinity for mineralocorticoid receptors as aldosterone; excess cortisol (as seen with chronic liquorice ingestion) binds to and activates mineralocorticoid receptors in the kidney that cause sodium retention and potassium excretion, producing an increased extracellular volume (resulting in raised blood pressure) and hypokalaemia (resulting in weakness and muscle spasm).

Some plants contain compounds with oestrogenic effects. The isoflavone genistein, which is found in soy beans, is probably the most widely studied but the most potent is 8-prenyl naringenin which is found in hops. These compounds antagonize oestrogen in some tissues yet express oestrogenic activity in other tissues. This is because they bind to the two different types of oesstrogen receptor (OR) with varying affinities. They generally have low affinity for the classical OR-α but bind with almost similar affinity to oestradiol to the OR-β receptor. Expression of the two OR subtypes varies across tissues. The classical receptor OR-α is distributed across reproductive cells, especially those of the breast and uterus, whereas OR-β is found mainly in brain, bone, bladder and vascular endothelium. It has been proposed that phytoestrogens may have potentially protective effects against mammary cancer, prostatic cancer, osteoporosis and atherosclerosis. The evidence is based mainly on experiments in animals which have been fed on large amounts of soy isoflavones. There is no direct evidence in humans. While claims are being made for the health effects of soy isoflavones, the safety of these compounds is now an issue of intense scrutiny by regulatory bodies. Of particular concern is the relatively high exposure of infants to phytoestrogens in soy-based breastmilk substitutes, which may influence the hormonal balance in later life.

■ 10.2.2 MYCOTOXINS

Mycotoxins are products of filamentous fungi that grow particularly on grains, seeds, nuts and dried fruit. In developed countries routine surveillance of mycotoxins on the import of potentially contaminated materials, use of fungicides and good storage conditions minimizes exposure to mycotoxins. Aflatoxins are a naturally occurring family of mycotoxin produced mainly by *Aspergillus flavus*, which grows on grains and nuts, especially peanuts, and thrives in hot and humid climates. At least 13 different types of aflatoxin have been identified, with aflatoxin B1 considered to be the most toxic. Aflatoxin B1 is one of the most potent carcinogens known to humans and the levels in foods are regularly monitored in the European community to ensure they do not exceed 2 μg/kg grain. Peanuts and dried apricots are the foods most often found to be contaminated with aflatoxins. Humans metabolize aflatoxin B1 to an 8, 9-epoxide in the liver which can form DNA adducts and result in liver cancer. Several other mycotoxins produced by other fungi are also monitored such as patulin (contaminates apple juice – can cause liver damage and haemorrhaging), ochratoxin A (contaminates cereals and coffee – can cause kidney damage), trichothenes (contaminates cereals – can cause bone marrow damage) and zearalenone (contaminates maize – has oestrogenic effects).

Mycotoxins are produced under conditions of warmth and humidity by fungi growing on nuts and grains. Aflatoxin B1 can cause liver cancer

■ 10.2.3 MARINE TOXINS

Algal toxins that accumulate in the marine food chain are a significant hazard for some fish-eating populations. Ciguatera is a sporadic form of human poisoning caused by the consumption of contaminated subtropical and tropical marine finfish (barracuda, grouper, snappers and mackerel) that causes neuropathy and paralysis and can be fatal. It is estimated that there are approximately 30,000 cases/year in the world, mainly in the Pacific and Caribbean. Ciguatoxin is produced by the dinoflagellate *Gambierdiscus toxicus* and accumulates in the flesh and viscera of fish. The toxin is a potent sodium channel blocker.

A related toxin (tetrodoxin) is responsible for fugu or balloon fish poisoning. Tetrodoxin is an extremely potent sodium channel blocker (10 μg/kg body weight is toxic) and one fish contains enough tetrodoxin to kill about 30 people. In Japan, where the fish is consumed as a delicacy, there are specially trained and licensed fugu chefs who are specially trained to remove the poisonous parts. However, deaths still occur. From 1974 to 1983 there were 646 reported cases of fugu fish-poisoning in Japan, with 179 fatalities. It is a continuing problem in Japan, with between 30 and 100 cases of poisoning reported every year, although most of these cases are caused by home preparation. In China deaths have occurred where fugu fish have been inadvertently mixed with other processed fish.

Dinoflagellate algae have long been known to cause red tides in the Pacific and they can affect waters around the British Isles between the months of May and August. The dinoflagellate *Gonyaulax catanella* produces a toxin called saxitoxin which is a potent neurotoxin. Shellfish which filter the dinoflagellates accumulate the toxin. Related toxins cause diarrhetic shellfish poisoning and amnesic shellfish poisoning. Monitoring programmes minimize exposure of the population to these algal toxins by placing controls on the sale of shellfish from affected areas. Amnesic shellfish poisoning was first reported in Canada but has since been reported in Europe and Japan. Global warming may change the geographical distribution of algal blooms. It is also possible that toxin-producing algae are spread by the discharge of bilge water from ships. As contaminated shellfish could be imported from countries where marine toxicoses are prevalent, it has become essential for food importers to be able to identify the source of origin of shellfish.

Algal blooms can produce toxins that accumulate in seafood

■ 10.3 CONTAMINANTS

The development of increasingly sensitive methods of analysis has focused attention on the presence of many harmful or potentially harmful substances in the environment, which may be present in minute amounts in foods. These may be held to render the food harmful to health or unfit for consumption but the assessment will again be a matter for judgment or opinion. All human activity carries risk, against this must be offset the benefit. For example, the use of pesticides and fertilizers offers stability of food supply but on the other hand they may harm health.

■ 10.3.1 PESTICIDES, FUNGICIDES, HERBICIDES AND FERTILIZERS

A large array of chemicals are used in modern food production and they have been responsible for increased yields of food and decreasing post-harvest losses. Foodborne exposure to agricultural and environmental chemicals results in much public concern in the UK. Owing to exquisitely sensitive methods of detection, trace amounts of potentially harmful chemicals can be detected in many foods. However, the levels of human exposure to these chemicals are generally well below the tolerable daily intakes in the UK. In most developed countries the use and application of agrochemicals is carefully regulated, monitored and reviewed and the generally held view is that the appropriate use of agrochemicals in food production is not a significant hazard to human health.

However, these chemicals are not always used appropriately, especially in less economically developed countries, where safety standards are not rigorously applied. Thus pesticides which are banned in economically developed countries (e.g. DDT) may still be used to control the spread of insect-borne diseases such as malaria.

Most agrochemicals are toxic to humans, e.g. organophosphates can cause nerve damage, and some are potentially carcinogenic (atrazine, phenoxy acid herbicides, 2, 4, 5-T, lindane, methoxychlor and toxaphene). The levels of agrochemicals in food are well below those likely to cause harm and the main hazards are to people working with them. However, some agrochemicals are not readily excreted from the body and are able to accumulate in tissues, especially fatty tissues, and so low intakes could be cumulatively toxic. The use of such persistent compounds is being phased out and foods are regularly monitored to ensure that maximum residue levels in foods are not exceeded. Monitoring of levels of pesticides in body fat has shown that the levels are steadily falling in the UK.

Large amounts of nitrates are used as fertilizers throughout the world. Nitrates are very water soluble and excessive use of nitrates can pollute water supplies. There are now controls to ensure levels of nitrates in drinking water do not exceed 50 mg/l. However, certain vegetables such as iceberg lettuce and spinach accumulate nitrate. A survey published in 2001 showed these vegetables contained on average about 3,000 mg/kg. The acceptable daily intake for nitrate is 3.65 mg/kg body weight which is equivalent to 219 mg/day for a 60 kg person and this amount is often exceeded by vegetarians who consume large amounts of vegetables.

Nitrate is regarded as relatively non-toxic but nitrite which can be derived from nitrate is regarded as toxic. Nitrate can be converted to nitrite by bacteria and this can happen during fermentation of food, e.g. pickling, as well as in the stomach when acidity is low. Saltpetre (potassium nitrate) has long been used to make salted meats such as bacon and ham. In this reaction, nitrate is reduced to nitrite and reacts with myoglobin to give a pink compound which gives ham and bacon their characteristic colour. In the body, a similar reaction occurs if the gastric acidity is low (e.g. in infants) permitting bacterial growth. Nitrite is formed, absorbed and competes with oxygen for binding to haemoglobin with the subsequent formation of methaemoglobin. If excessive amounts of methaemoglobin are formed it impairs the oxygen carrying capacity and the infant appears blue (hence the term blue baby syndrome). This only occurs when intake of nitrate is high and there have been no reports in the UK since 1972.

Nitrites can also react with secondary amines and amides to form nitrosamines and nitrosamides, which are potent carcinogens. The consumption of salted pickled fish in China is associated with a high risk of nasogastric cancer and studies have shown the salted fish to contain N-nitrosodimethylamine which can cause cancer in animals. The level of nitrate in food does not appear to be a good predictor of nitrosamine formation. Furthermore, there appears to be no relationship between nitrate in food and drinking water and cancer risk in the UK.

Agricultural chemicals used in food pose little risk to health if used properly

■ 10.3.2 DIOXINS AND DIOXIN-LIKE POLYCHLORINATED BIPHENYLS (PCBS)

Dioxins are toxic substances produced during many industrial processes involving chlorine such as waste incineration, chemical and pesticide manufacturing and pulp and paper bleaching. They have no immediate effect on health, even at the highest levels found in foods, but potential risks to health come from long-term exposure to high levels. The most potent dioxin 2, 3, 7, 8-tetrachlorodibenzo-p-dioxin (TCCD) is a known human carcinogen and endocrine disruptor. TCCD is a ligand for the arylhydro-carbon (AhR) receptor and blocks the binding to OR-α. The toxicity of other dioxins and chemicals like PCBs that act like dioxin are measured in relation to TCDD in units called tetrachlorodibenzo-p-dioxin equivalents (TEQ) by comparing their relative binding to the AhR receptor. PCBs have been used since the early 1930s, mainly in electrical equipment such as coolants, but their manufacture and general use stopped in the 1970s. Nevertheless, substantial amounts of PCBs have been released into the environment. Both dioxins and dioxin-like PCBs are persistent organic pollutants that degrade only slowly and so are widespread in the environment and accumulate in the food chain. Dioxins deposited on plants can be taken up by animals and aquatic organisms and concentrated into the food chain so that animals have higher concentrations. Within animals, dioxins tend to accumulate in fat, especially in the liver. About 95 per cent of the average person's exposure to dioxins occurs through consumption of food, especially food containing animal fat. Levels of dioxins in the diet have fallen over the past ten years and the World Health Organisation has recommended that the Tolerable Daily Intake for dioxins and dioxin-like PCBs should be below 2 pg TEQ/kg body weight/d. Yet the amounts supplied by breast milk to infants in the UK are 170 pg TEQ/kg body weight/d which is considerably in excess of the recommendations. However, the benefits of breastfeeding are believed to far outweigh the hypothetical risk from short term exposure dioxins.

Dioxins and PCBs are persistent environmental pollutants that accumulate in animal fat. The hazards they pose with regard to risk of human cancer remains largely hypothetical

■ 10.3.3 MICROBIOLOGICAL CONTAMINATION

Microbiological contamination of food and water is the main cause of diarrhoea, which contributes to causing about 3 million deaths among children under five (mainly in developing countries). The effects of foodborne infection are not restricted to the gastrointestinal tract, as illustrated by viral hepatitis, tuberculosis and haemolytic-uraemic syndrome caused by *E.coli* 0157. Foodborne parasitic diseases are also a major public health problem in developing countries, but not in developed countries.

The *USA National Food Safety Initiative* attributes 9,000 deaths and between 6.5 and 33 million episodes of illness annually to foodborne microbial illness. In England and Wales, 300 deaths and 35,000 hospital admissions are attributed annually to infectious gastrointestinal diseases. Laboratory reports indicate that campylobacter, salmonella, rotavirus A and small round structured virus are the most commonly detected pathogens. Surveillance reports underestimate the true incidence of infectious gastrointestinal disease by two orders of magnitude; it is estimated that there are 9.4 million cases of infectious gastrointestinal disease in England each year.

The emergence of new foodborne pathogens such as *E.coli* 0157, which has been detected in the faeces of up to 15 per cent of British cattle, is of particular concern as beef is often consumed undercooked or rare. Intensive poultry production is linked to the epidemic of *Salmonella enteritidis* phage type 4 that has emerged in the UK, Europe and the USA. *S.enteritidis* can be detected in 1 per cent of eggs and in about one fifth of all poultry. Raw or unpasteurized milk and eggs are a significant cause of food poisoning

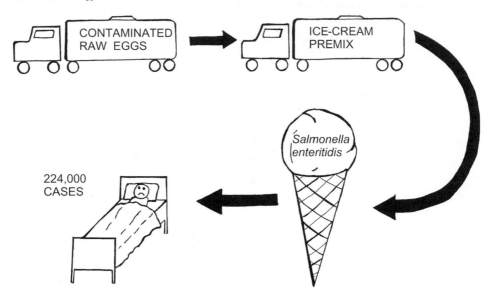

• **Figure 10.1** Pandemic of food poisoning caused by contamination of ice-cream premix by transport in a tanker that previously had contained raw egg white

in both the UK and USA (Figure 10.1). Providing poultry and eggs are cooked properly, the risk of food poisoning is low. Poor food hygiene and inadequate processing, particularly within the home, contribute to causing infectious intestinal disease but cannot be blamed for food poisoning outbreaks associated with shellfish, especially molluscs which are particularly linked to viral infections.

Microbiological contamination of food is a major public health problem and new antibiotic resistant organisms are rapidly spreading as a result of globalization of the food trade

The continued use of antibiotics as growth promoters for poultry and pigs is of concern because it has resulted in the emergence of multi-drug resistant strains of pathogenic bacteria such as quinolone resistant *Campylobacter jejuni* and *Salmonella enterica* serotype tymphomurium DT104. The sewage sludge generated from intensive poultry and pig meat production might be an important origin for the spread of antibiotic resistant genes and pathogenic bacteria into the food chain.

■ 10.3.4 TRANSMISSIBLE SPONGIFORM ENCEPHALOPATHIES

Transmissible spongiform encephalopathies (TSE) are a class of disease which can be transmitted by feeding on brain and nervous tissues, generally within a species. They can also be transmitted both within and between species by contaminated surgical instruments. The first recorded outbreak of TSE in humans was reported in Papua New Guinea in the 1950s among the Fore tribe who practised a form of ritual cannabalism of the dead. The disease (known as kuru) resulted in a progressive neurological disorder and the brain had a spongiform appearance. The causative agent is believed to be a protein like material called a prion, which can self-replicate. Prions are proteins that are found in the brains of both normal and afflicted individuals. Prion proteins are found in two forms, the wild type form (PrPc) and the mutant form (PrPsc). It has been hypothesized that a mutant prion protein acts as a chaperone, causing incorrect folding of wild type prion proteins. In other words, mutant prion proteins self-propagate: incorrectly folded proteins lead

• **Figure 10.2** Bovine spongiform encephalopathy in cattle and possible modes of transmission

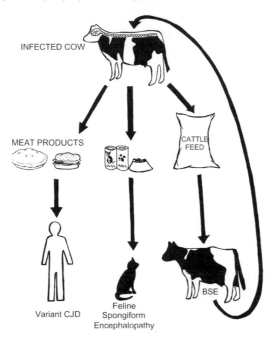

INFECTED COW

MEAT PRODUCTS

CATTLE FEED

Variant CJD

Feline Spongiform Encephalopathy

BSE

to more incorrectly folded proteins. The mutant proteins have a tendency to aggregate, giving rise to characteristic rod like plaques in brain tissue. This in turn results in the death of the brain tissue giving it a spongy appearance.

An epidemic of bovine spongiform encephalopathy (BSE) emerged in dairy cattle in the UK from 1986, peaking in 1992 when 1,000 cases a month were being reported. BSE apparently arose because brain tissue from cattle and sheep was being fed to dairy cattle as a protein supplement. Scrapie is a form of TSE found in sheep that has been present in the UK for over fifty years and it was suggested that BSE arose from infected sheep offal. However, it appears that BSE is more likely to have had its origin in cattle. In 1988, a ban on the use of the bovine and ovine offal for use in the diets of ruminants came into place and the incidence of BSE in younger cattle started to fall. However, cattle previously infected with the offal continued to develop the disease. Cattle do not generally show clinical signs of the disease until at least 3 years after exposure.

In 1996 a new form of TSE was reported in young people and was called variant Creutzfeldt-Jakob disease (vCJD). This is a progressive disease that results in paralysis and death. By August 2002 a total of 115 people had contracted the disease. It seems almost certain that vCJD was transmitted to humans from cattle with BSE, as a similar prion pattern is found in humans and in cattle with BSE and in cats and mice transfected with BSE. The exact mode of transmission remains uncertain, i.e. it is uncertain whether it occurred from transmissions resulting from the consumption of packets of infective material in foods such as beefburgers or whether it was transmitted parenterally from medical products such as vaccines made with infected bovine material. Cattle with clinical signs of BSE have been removed from the food chain since 1988, and additional precautions were taken to remove potentially infective offal from healthy animals since 1989; since

1996 controls have been tightened with only cattle below 30 months entering the food chain, with the exception of some herds which have never received feed concentrates. The final number of people likely to be infected by the disease is uncertain as it may take 10–15 years following exposure to develop. Pessimistic estimates suggested that tens of thousands would be affected but more realistic estimates suggest the numbers will be in the hundreds.

Globalization of the food trade has meant that BSE has spread to other countries in Europe as well as to the Middle East and Japan. The United States has banned the use of blood products from people who have resided in the UK for fear that it may lead to an epidemic of vCJD in the USA. The probability of transmission of vCJD by blood is very low but in this case the USA have applied the precautionary principle which is defined as follows: 'When an activity raises threats of harm to human health or the environment, precautionary measures should be taken even if some cause-and-effect relationships are not fully established scientifically.' The BSE episode particularly illustrates the need to assess risks to human health from changes in farming practices.

Transmissible encephalopathies such as BSE can be transmitted between species by feeding on infected brain and spinal cord

■ 10.4 FOOD ADDITIVES

The benefits of modern food processing are often taken for granted: increased food availability, decreased cost and greater convenience. Food processing is essential to feed a large urban population: it destroys naturally occurring toxicants and inhibits the growth and spread of pathogenic and spoilage organisms. Food processing also necessitates the use of food additives to act as preservatives, as processing aids, and to replace colour and nutrients lost during processing. The safety and use of food additives is strictly controlled by legislation. Food additives are compounds that are intentionally added to food for a particular purpose and have to be shown to be safe before they can be used. For example, the sweetener aspartame is methyl-aspartyl-phenylalanine. It is about 100 times sweeter than sugar and is used in low calorie drinks at a level of about 500 mg/l. On digestion it is broken down to its constituent amino acids, aspartic acid and phenylalanine, and small amounts of methanol. Before aspartame was approved it had to undergo a battery of toxicological tests in both animals and humans to show that it was safe.

Food additives are intentionally added to food to make it safer, look better and to improve food quality. They have to be shown to be safe, effective and necessary before they are approved

The permitted list of additives in Europe are given E numbers to signify that they have been approved for use in all countries in the European Union. The additives on the permitted list are reviewed every five years or so and if new information suggests an additive has undesirable effects it is removed from the list. Allegations frequently reported in the media that food additives are a major cause of food allergy and hyperactivity have never been substantiated.

■ 10.5 NEW DEVELOPMENTS

An improved understanding of the molecular basis for non-communicable diseases has led to opportunities to design foods that have health promoting effects. Advances in biotechnology have also meant that it is possible to modify existing foods in a way that may influence their health promoting properties. With the unravelling of the human genome and the identification of common gene polymorphisms, in the future we may be able to design diets that are appropriate for an individual's genotype.

■ **10.5.1 FUNCTIONAL FOODS**

The term functional food is used to describe specific beneficial effects resulting from the consumption of foods and their constituents upon physiological or psychological functions or biological activities but do not include nutrient function claims. Such claims might include risk reduction (e.g. 'helps lower blood cholesterol') or improvement of a function (e.g. 'helps rehydration') or modification or preservation of health (e.g. 'helps maintain a healthy gut flora'). The position of these claims in law is in limbo as explicit health claims are currently forbidden in the European Union but are permitted in some other countries such as the USA and Japan. However, there is an increasing number of foods making implied health claims and some are clearly fraudulent. Legislation is being considered at the European level to regulate such claims. Some examples of functional foods that have a good molecular basis for their action are given below.

- Plant phytosterols and phytostanols are added to margarine, yoghurt and milk and actively lower blood LDL cholesterol concentrations on average by 10 per cent with an intake of 2–3 g/d. These compounds competitively inhibit the absorption of cholesterol, which is provided by the diet or secreted in bile.
- An important discovery made in the 1960s was that small amounts of sugar and salt enhance the absorption of water from the small intestine because they stimulate active transport processes. Simple oral rehydration solutions are widely used for rehydrating people with diarrhoea. They typically contain 3.5 g/l NaCl, 2.5 g/l NaHCO$_3$ and 20 g/l glucose. The food industry has cashed in on this idea in designing sports drinks that cause more rapid rehydration than ordinary beverages such as cola and fruit juice.
- Probiotics are the lactic acid bacteria and bifidobacteria which are widely used in yoghurts and other dairy products. Prebiotics are non-digestible food ingredients such as fructo-oligosaccharides and lactose which selectively stimulate the growth or activities, or both, of lactobacilli or bifidobacteria in the colon. In breastfed infants, the large intestine is colonized by bifidobacteria, whose growth is stimulated by lactose in breast milk, and this helps to act as a barrier against infection by pathogenic bacteria. It is believed that the use of pre- and probiotics by adults may help maintain a healthy gut microbial flora. Probiotics have been used to treat travellers' diarrhoea.
- Some sugar alcohols such as xylitol and palatinose are used to make 'tooth friendly' confectionery. They are not fermented in the mouth and inhibit the growth of the bacteria that cause tooth decay.

■ **10.6 GENETICALLY MODIFIED FOOD**

Recombinant DNA technology can be used to genetically modify foods in ways that were not previously possible with conventional breeding. Traits can be selected and transferred across species. To date, only a few foods that have been genetically modified using recombinant DNA technology have been approved for food use. Food ingredients, such as amino acids and vitamins, as well as enzymes from genetically modified (GM) microorganisms have been widely used in the food industry. For example, in the UK most cheese is made with chymosin, which is made by GM yeast, rather than from rennet, which is prepared from the stomachs of new born calves. A significant number of crops have been genetically modified and are widely grown in the USA, Argentina, Canada and China. In 2001, over 37 million hectares in the USA were planted with GM crops. From 1996 to 2001, herbicide tolerance has consistently been the most sought-after trait with insect resistance second.

Insect pest resistance is engineered into crops by taking the gene for *Bacillus thurungiensis* toxin (BT) and transfecting it into plants such as maize and cotton. This makes the crop resistant to lepidopteran pests such as the European corn borer and the boll weevil. BT toxin is harmless to humans. Herbicide tolerance is engineered into crops by transfecting plants with genes for proteins that detoxify specific herbicides (such as glyphosate, glufosinate, bromoxynil and sulfonylurea). For example, the herbicide glyphosate (marketed as Roundup™) blocks the enzyme 3-enolpyruvylshikimate-5-phosphate synthase (EPSPS). Resistance to glyphosate is engineered into a plant by adding a gene from a soil bacterium (*Agrobacterium* spp.) that encodes a glyphosate-resistant version of the EPSPS enzyme, to make the plants resistant to the herbicide. Herbicide resistant crops require less chemical treatments than traditional crops to control weeds and this can result in less soil erosion if the herbicide is used immediately prior to the emergence of the seedling. These modifications decrease the input of agrochemicals into food production and save the farmer money. However, they do not result in increased yields or improvements in nutritional quality or taste and consumers have yet to be convinced of the benefits of GM crops.

GM crops can be developed to be drought or frost resistant or to have altered nutritional value. It is also possible to modify the fatty acid composition of oilseed rape. However, the only GM modified oilseed rape in commercial production is one with a higher saturated fatty acid content (high laurate canola oil). Animals can also be genetically modified to grow faster or can be cloned so that production characteristics are maintained. However, there is considerable opposition to the use of GM for animal production from environmental and animal rights groups and there is likely to be a moratorium in this area for at least the next five years in view of the current lack of consumer confidence in biotechnology.

While the genetic modification of food at first sight offers a number of potential benefits, the safety assessment of GM foods poses a new challenge. The classical toxicological approach used for chemicals, which involves feeding animals intakes 100 times the amounts likely to be consumed by humans to demonstrate toxic effects, is not appropriate when applied to foods that may contribute up to 20 per cent of the dietary intake. The approach taken by the UK Advisory Committee on Novel Foods and Processes in assessing the safety of GM foods has been to consider each food on a case-by-case basis, to ensure that there are no hazards associated with the method used to transfer the gene, that the genetic modification is stable, that the processing of the food denatures the DNA, that there are no new allergens, and that the GM food is substantially equivalent in terms of chemical composition to the unmodified parent organism. Despite negative reports in the media, no adverse reactions in humans to approved GM foods have yet been reported. However, it will be some years until we can be certain that there are no adverse effects.

SUMMARY

- Adverse reactions are usually idiosyncratic and may be caused by allergy to proteins in food, particularly nuts and shellfish, or by bioactive compounds in food.
- Naturally occurring toxicants are a much greater risk to health than artificial contaminants especially in developing countries.
- The centralization and globalization of food makes the risks of large-scale outbreaks of food poisoning more likely.
- Genetic modification of food offers potential benefits because it decreases the amount of chemicals used in food production.

■ FINAL REMARKS AND CONCLUSION

Advances in technology have enabled world food supply to keep pace with population growth. We also now understand more of the molecular basis of nutritional deficiencies and the role of diet in non-communicable disease. For the first time in the history of the world, there are more overweight people than undernourished people; however, they live in different countries. As the world population is forecast to double over the next fifty years, food production must continue to increase to meet the needs of people in developing countries. The availability of water is a major constraint on food production in those countries and efforts will be needed to conserve water for food production. Biotechnology may have a role in achieving the goal of sustainable development, which recognizes the need for technology without environmental damage. An efficient food industry and distribution system can also decrease waste. However, the food industry cannot be allowed to be unfettered and it is the role of government to ensure that industry applies proper risk assessment and management procedures, that independent surveillance and monitoring occurs and that there are internationally agreed food standards. Education is also needed to alert consumers to risks from food and how to minimize them. Finally, we still have much to learn regarding the molecular basis of human nutrition and we need to be prepared to change our views as new evidence emerges.

FURTHER READING

Sanders, T.A. (1999) 'Food production and food safety', *BMJ*, 318: 1689–93.
Buttriss, J. (2002) *British Nutrition Foundation: Adverse Reactions to Food.* Oxford: Blackwell Scientific Press.
Center for Food Safety and Applied Nutrition Foodborne Pathogenic Microorganisms and Natural Toxins Handbook. http://www.cfsan.fda.gov/~mow/intro.html (accessed 12/2/03).

INDEX